Make Over Your Metabolism

by
Robert Reames

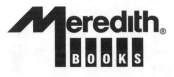

Meredith Books
1716 Locust Street
Des Moines, Iowa 50309–3023
www.meredithbooks.com

First Edition. Printed in the United States of America.
Library of Congress Control Number: 2005931898
ISBN: 0-696-23055-0

See Your Doctor First

This diet and fitness book is designed to provide helpful information on the subjects addressed. This book is sold with the understanding that the author and publisher are not rendering medical, health, or other personal services. The suggestions for specific exercise routines, foods, and lifestyle recommendations are not intended to replace medical advice or treatment by your physician. All questions and concerns regarding your health, metabolism, weight, nutrition, and physical activity should be directed to your physician, particularly if you have any health problems or medical problems (including if you are pregnant or lactating). All reasonable attempts have been made to include the most recent and factual research and medical reports regarding exercise and nutrition. However, there is no guarantee that future research, particularly human studies, will not change the information presented here. Further, the internet addresses in this book were accurate at the time of printing. Individual needs vary, and no nutrition or exercise program will meet everyone's needs. Be sure to consult your physician prior to following any of the suggestions presented in this book and also before changing your diet or exercise routine. You should rely on your physician's advice regarding whether the suggestions presented in this book are appropriate for you, and you should rely on your physician to establish your weight goal. The author and publisher disclaim all liability associated with the recommendations and guidelines set forth in this book.

Robert Reames, CSCS, *D, CN, RTS1, CPT

Born and raised in Indiana and a firm believer in hard work, dedication, and honoring commitments, Robert Reames brings to his clients nationwide more than 20 years of experience in the areas of health, fitness, nutrition, and wellness. His strong athletic background and the fact that he was overweight as a child continue to fuel his passion for both one-on-one training, group training, and consulting as well as presentations on the entire spectrum of the world of health.

Upon his graduation from Ball State University, Robert ventured West to continue his education and obtained his strength, conditioning, and nutrition certifications from well-respected organizations in the health, fitness, and nutrition industries. His certifications include Certified Strength and Conditioning Specialist (recertified with distinction) from the National Strength and Conditioning Association; Certified Personal Trainer (advanced level) from the National Academy of Sports Medicine; Certified Nutritionist from American Health Science University; Resistance Training Specialist from Resistance University; and Medical Exercise Specialist from the American Academy of Health, Fitness, and Rehabilitation Professionals. He is also a professional member of the International Association of Fitness Professionals, the National Strength and Conditioning Association, and the American College of Sports Medicine. Robert believes strongly that continuing his education in this vast field is a lifelong endeavor that provides his viewers and clientele with the latest in exercise science as well as the most current information in the fields of health, wellness, exercise, nutrition, weight/fat loss, antiaging, sports-specific training, and injury prevention.

Robert is currently in his third season as the official trainer and fitness consultant for the *Ultimate Weight Loss Challenge* on the nationally syndicated television program *Dr. Phil*. He has appeared as an exercise consultant on the KTLA *Morning Show*, Discovery Channel's FitTV, QVC, and as a member of the Extreme Team on ABC's *Extreme Makeover*. Robert hosts the highly acclaimed *Extreme Makeover Weight Loss for Beginners* DVD, which is distributed by Buena Vista Home Entertainment. He continues to make appearances in both television and radio for local and regional talk, news, and variety shows. He also does many live presentations and speaking engagements. Robert has contributed or been featured in many national magazines, including *Fitness, E Pregnancy, Family Circle, Prevention, Self, Sonik, Sweat, Oxygen,* and Dr. Phil's *Next Level*. His articles appear on www.drphil.com, in "Advice from the Experts" on www.precor.com, and on www.miowatch.com representing the MIO heart rate monitor.

Robert continues to train and consult individuals from every walk of life. With a lifelong commitment to the fields of health, fitness, nutrition, wellness, and education—and given a person's own genetic window of opportunity—Robert helps people be the best that they can be!

Acknowledgments

The *Make Over Your Metabolism* program provides a "road map" to permanent weight loss. I want to help you accomplish realistic goals and be the healthiest individual you can be. My mission is to eliminate the confusion that you have heard over the years and give you information based on proven science. You can put these ideas to work in your life to bring you to—and help you surpass—these goals and forever maintain the highest level of health that you desire. This is not a temporary plan. Temporary plans yield temporary results. This is a toolbox from which to draw every day and which will help you succeed for the duration of your long life. Whether very fit or an eager beginner, may you continue to rise to your top level—your "personal best"—and achieve the great health that you deserve both for yourself and your loved ones.

Thank you to my wife, Arminae, and my daughter, Audrey. You both are my true inspiration and two of the strongest women I'll ever know. I thank God for every day of my life with you. I am whole because you both are in my life. Thank you for your support, your love, and our family. I love you so much, and I am truly a blessed man.

To my mother, Audrey, "Grandma Audrey," and my father, Bill: Ma, thanks for your love, support, and bringing out the best in me. I can always count on you, and I want to thank you most for teaching me the importance of being a good and loving person. And Pa, I wish you were here. We miss you so much. You left this earth way too early. But I feel you walk with me every day. You both "raised me right" and I feel you in my heart and soul every day. Thank you for the opportunities that you have always provided to me. I appreciate you both more than you could ever know. I love you both so much.

To Dr. Phil and Robin McGraw: Phil, "thank you" cannot begin to convey my appreciation for the opportunities that you have provided to me. Bottom line: You put me on the national map and I am ever grateful to you. To work on your team and be the official trainer for the most successful weight loss movement of our time is a great honor. I remember so well more than three years ago reading *Self Matters* and your 10 "Life Laws" in *Life Strategies*. Your teachings continue to enhance both my personal and professional lives and encourage me to attain my own personal best. American and international television is blessed to have you. To have had this opportunity to know you and work with both you and Robin personally is awesome and a true blessing. Robin, thank you for your unwavering support. You are an outstanding role model for women, and your wisdom on life is unparalleled. You are both incredible human beings and truly phenomenal athletes! I am truly grateful for your friendship and to be part of your team.

To the staff of the *Dr. Phil* show, Jaime Geffner, Carla Pennington, Scott Madsen, Jill Skinner, Judy Rybak, David Goldman, Sarah Gebeke, Eric Streit, Chandler Hayes, Louis DiCenzo, Lisa Williams, John Heinz, Cari Felson, Bill Vosburgh, Alan Bosshardt, Annette Jones, and every single member of the staff: You are not only amazing people but quite obviously the best and most consummate professionals working in all of television today. I absolutely love working with you all!

Special thanks to all of the participants over the years on the *Ultimate Weight Loss Challenge*. You continue to bring out the best in me, and it's awesome to see you all inspire the world with your personal success on Dr. Phil McGraw's program. Thanks especially to Jim Toth, Monika Barkley, Judith and Janice Blowe, and the Pennington family for your contributions to this book.

Thanks and much love to my mother-in-law, Hasmick, and my father-in-law, Ham—"Mama Jan and Papa Jan." You are great teachers for how to live a healthy life. And thank you for bringing your daughter Arminae into this world. And to my sister-in-law, Seda—"Cookie." What can I say? You are like a sister to me. The world has only begun to benefit from your gifts.

To my friend, my leader on this book, and the top agent in the galaxy, Matthew Guma and Inkwell Management. You orchestrated this entire production from the get-go. I knew five seconds into our first phone conversation that you were the perfect agent for me. What an education you have given me. Thanks for your knowledge, your friendship, your camaraderie, and your leadership. And thank you for understanding the great value in my message from the beginning and helping me bring this forth to America. You're awesome!

Thanks to Justin Larry Loeber and Tracy Behar for connecting me with Matthew Guma and Inkwell!

To my friend Dr. Maggie Greenwood-Robinson, who is undisputedly this nation's top nutritionist and health, fitness, and nutrition writer. Thank you so much for all you have taught me, for your passion, your leadership, your guidance, and your dedication to this work. It clearly would not be the book it is without you. It was an amazing experience working on this book, and I greatly appreciate the opportunity to work with you.

To my in-house editor at Meredith Books, Stephanie Karpinske, and my art director, Chad Jewell. Thank you both for your commitment in the making of *Make Over Your Metabolism*. Your incredible talent, attention to detail, and your magnificent creative vision have made this book the best that it can be. You are the very best, and I am so very grateful to both of you.

Many, many special thanks to Linda Cunningham of Meredith Books. Linda, you are phenomenal. You understood from the onset that America did not need yet another weight loss gimmick, but rather a "road map" to help conquer the fight with obesity and achieve optimum health. You are the best in the industry, and I am inspired and fortunate to be working for you. Thank you to Amy Nichols, Gina Rickert, and Steve Rogers. I am so appreciative to you and the entire Meredith staff. You are all consummate professionals and wonderful people. The good Lord most definitely directed me to the right place.

Thanks to the nation's best manager, my great friend Cat Josell, for your guidance and wisdom, and for putting together the awesome team for me. I love working with you! Chris Trela, Babette Perry, Carole Bruckner, and Jason Pinyan at ICM—you all rock! And thanks to Traci Harper, publicist extraordinaire. From the "rock 'n' roll aerobics days" to now you've been a great support and friend.

To my brother John for being the godfather of our precious Audrey. Thanks for all your legal help, but more important, thanks for being my second-best friend (next to Arminae) and a positive role model for me. Thanks to my sister Mare and my brother Steve for being so great. And thank you for your ever encouraging words and showing me at a very young age the power of a caring spirit.

Thanks to an outstanding photographer, Andy Lyons, and photo assistant, Adam Albright. Thank you to hair and makeup artist, Lesa Courter, and to Shanaz for great haircuts. And thanks to Heather Knochenmus, the model in this book, and to The Suites of 800 Locust for the use of your fitness center.

Thank you to my friends Oleg Bouimer and Yulin Zhao for your friendship and incredible ability to heal. Thanks to Shawn Nelson for your continuing work with me. Thanks to Deborah Robinson for always being willing to "talk shop." And thanks to my wonderful friend J. J. Virgin for your help, your valuable influence on me as a professional, and your contribution to *Make Over Your Metabolism*.

Thank you to all of my key clients over the years and to Jay Roth, Tom Freston, Michael and Margo O'Connell, Cara Esposito, and Sara Kane for sharing your stories as part of this book. You have all helped me to develop as a professional and I appreciate all of your many years of support.

Thank you to my great friend and comrade Danny Valdez for your friendship over the years. You are the earth's most knowledgeable person on the full spectrum of the exercise equipment industry. And thanks to my friend Mike Dworkin for your support and friendship over the years.

My thanks to the National Strength and Conditioning Association (NSCA), National Academy of Sports Medicine (NASM), American Health Science University, and American College of Sports Medicine (ACSM) for your continuing education and providing me and health and fitness professionals everywhere with the latest in research and educational opportunity. And thank you especially to the NSCA for the personal support you have given to my work.

This book is dedicated to
my wife, Arminae, and my daughter, Audrey—the two pillars of
strength in my life. And my mother, Audrey, and late father,
Bill, who laid the foundation for who I am today.

MAKE OVER YOUR METABOLISM

Table of Contents

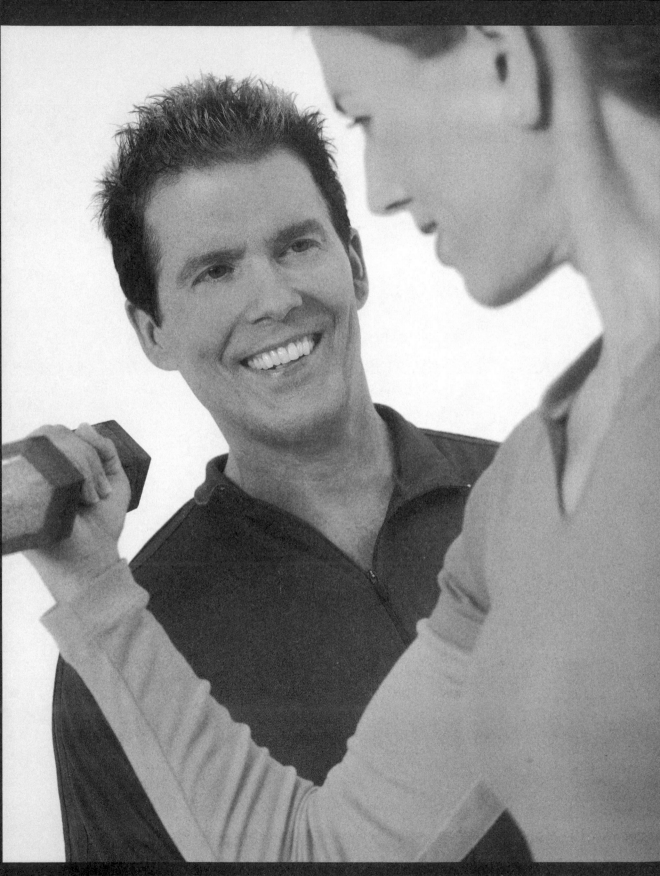

IF YOU'RE ON A MISSION TO SHED EXCESS POUNDS, LOSE INCHES, AND CHANGE THE WAY YOU LOOK, ONCE AND FOR ALL, THEN I'M YOUR GUY AND THIS IS YOUR PROGRAM. IN FACT THE *Make Over Your Metabolism* PROGRAM IS GOING TO BE THE easiest fitness program you've ever followed.

I mean really easy.

Here is why: You will learn an exercise method that requires no more than three hours a week but stimulates your body to burn the optimum amount of fat 24 hours a day, seven days a week—even on Sundays and legal holidays! While you're working, watching TV, and even sleeping, you will be on a continual fat burn because this program will keep your metabolism in sync day in and day out. On my program, you could be eating lunch right now but still burning calories because of the exercise you did two days ago!

You will also learn my Nutritional Life Plan that puts you in control of your food. This plan will show you that *what, when,* and *how often* you eat is vital for increasing your metabolism, maximizing your body's ability to burn fat, and taming cravings. I will also give you some little-known lifestyle tips that will help normalize your

I'm Your Personal Trainer

metabolism. These practices will not only help you lose weight but also make you feel energized and in much better health.

This is not hype, so please don't turn away thinking you've heard it all before. This is science-based truth. You can train your body to burn fat 24-7 and do it without hours of exhausting, muscle-wasting, time-consuming workouts.

People once thought any exercise that didn't have you running and sweating for hours upon hours wouldn't work well for fat loss. No more. Now we know how to get the maximum out of a workout for the minimal amount of time. As the saying goes, "It's about quality, not quantity." If you can devote just three hours each week to my special exercises, stick with my Nutritional Life Plan, and apply my fat-burn lifestyle tips, you *will* succeed and get a better body in an amazingly short time.

As you follow the *Make Over Your Metabolism* program, I will be with you every step of the way, guiding you with encouragement, inspiration, and motivation, just as I do with clients I work with in person. I've written this book so you'll feel like I'm right there with you, acting as your own personal trainer, someone who will help you realize all that you're capable of. I'll help you acknowledge all your progress and take pride in all your success, whether it's a 1-pound loss or a 5-pound one, a drop in your dress size or getting into that pair of jeans you've been wanting to put back on, or conquering that impulse to do nothing and hopping on the treadmill instead. I'll take you from potato chips and candy to fresh fruit and almonds. Together we are going to celebrate every single success in your life: the 30 minutes of exercising you put in, the healthy dinner you cook for yourself and your family, the new smaller-size outfit you buy, the moments you feel good about yourself because of what you've accomplished. I'll help you rise to the top of your game every time you step into that workout room.

Buying this book is like hiring me as a trainer in Los Angeles, but at a much more economical price. It's really an investment in you, and I appreciate that you have entrusted this part of your life to me because together we will do some great things.

I have designed this program for the millions of people who are intimidated by buff bodies and confused by what they see on exercise machine ads, in infomercials, in movies, and on magazine covers—all the airbrushed glitz and glamour paint unrealistic pictures for real people to try to emulate. They promote gimmicks that we all know will never work. Have you ever noticed that the more gimmicks that come out year after year, the fatter America gets? Many fitness magazines don't even speak to most Americans; they're largely fashion magazines with exercise pictures.

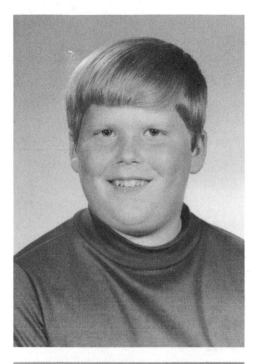

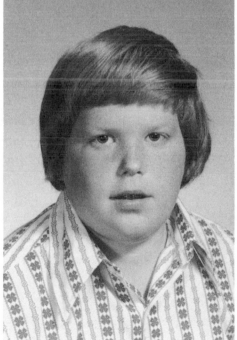

I was frequently teased and called "Fatso" as a child. These are my school pictures from grade 6 (above) and grade 8 (below). It was only after I got more involved in sports that the weight gradually came off.

When society and the media put a premium on having the "perfect body," it's tough to feel satisfied with how you look. You base your self-esteem on the girth of your thighs. You think you don't deserve to ever see your toes again. You're often fearful, and with good reason. You've been told you have to change, or else. You feel out of control, which only makes things worse. Frustration wins out and the goal is lost. That's why I'm glad you're holding this book in your hands. I want you to be the strongest, leanest, and best version of yourself. I want you to accomplish realistic goals, not try to live up to some standard from a picture of a model whose body has been perfected by a computer. This book is about performing at your best on any given day. It takes a simple yet effective—and time-efficient—approach to changing *your* body for the better and with it, your life. It's a program anyone can do, no matter what your fitness level, and one you'll want to stay with over time.

If you're wondering how a fitness guru could relate to what you're feeling, let me tell you a little bit about who I am and how I developed the *Make Over Your Metabolism* program. I was overweight as a kid, and my schoolmates in

Indiana called me "Fatso" and "Chubby." The teasing stung, but I hid the pain well. Underneath my happy-go-lucky personality, though, I was often mad and frustrated—so angry in fact that more than once I got into fights with kids who picked on me.

By junior high, I noticed girls. But they didn't notice me back, other than as a nice guy who was good at sports. I wanted to be popular with the girls and be the best athlete that I could be, so I started taking my conditioning drills for sports more seriously. I pulled way, way back on the pizza and fries. And the pounds came off. Finally the girls started noticing me.

In college I took jazz and other dance classes because I had aspirations of going into show business. But fate had other ideas! To stay in shape, I started taking aerobic dance classes. I was "discovered" by an aerobics instructor who asked me to start teaching classes—which I did the very next day! I am so grateful that I made that decision. My classes filled up and became very popular.

During those years I became determined to make a difference in people's lives by pursuing a career in health and fitness. To this day, the way I look and feel is a direct result of the way I live. As a husband and father, I want to take care of my health so my family always receives the best of me. It's very simple: To achieve long-term results, you must exercise regularly, consistently make the right food choices, and get proper rest.

The *Make Over Your Metabolism* program has thus grown out of my 20-plus years of working with all different kinds of clients—men, women, and kids at all weights and shapes who want to look great, feel great, and prolong their lives by developing healthier habits. I often work with busy executives who only have time to work out twice a week and, even then, may come in 15 or 20 minutes late due to their packed schedules. I'm obligated to give them their money's worth in the remaining time so they can achieve their goals. I've also trained people for television shows—a challenge that is full of deadlines—so I've helped people get in shape rapidly. One of my most rewarding jobs has been working with the *Dr. Phil* television show, particularly helping the "real people" participants on Dr. Phil's *Ultimate Weight Loss Challenge*. No matter who the client or what the circumstances, my job is all about getting results.

Over the years word has spread that my workouts are accessible, quick, efficient, and to the point—and that they work where other programs have failed. More people have started coming to me because they want to get the most results in the least amount of time. My clients are able to fit this program into their lives, and so can you.

The point of telling you my story is that I've been where you are today. And I'm here to tell you that your situation is not hopeless, not even close. You can and will succeed.

Your goal may simply be to reduce health risk factors so you can live to see your 5-year-old graduate from college. I applaud that goal. This book contains a realistic plan for real people. That means *you*—not the fallacy of the "best bodies of Hollywood." My passion is to teach people like you how to reach your physical potential and your highest fitness level. No matter what shape you are in, or what you have done in the past, you have the physical ability to succeed on this program.

I won't build on your fears; I will build on your passion to bring out the very best version of yourself.

- **You will become more active** than you ever thought possible, be able to move again, trim off fat and inches, and take control of the "fuel" that you put into your body.
- **You will start feeling good about yourself** again, and this will give you a newfound sense of control over your life.
- **Feelings of defeat will be wiped out** and replaced by the bright glow of victory.
- **Your shoulders will lift,** and you will walk toward the future with a new air of confidence and mastery.

You have it inside you to succeed; your abilities are just waiting to be developed. Now if you're ready—and I know you are—let's rock!

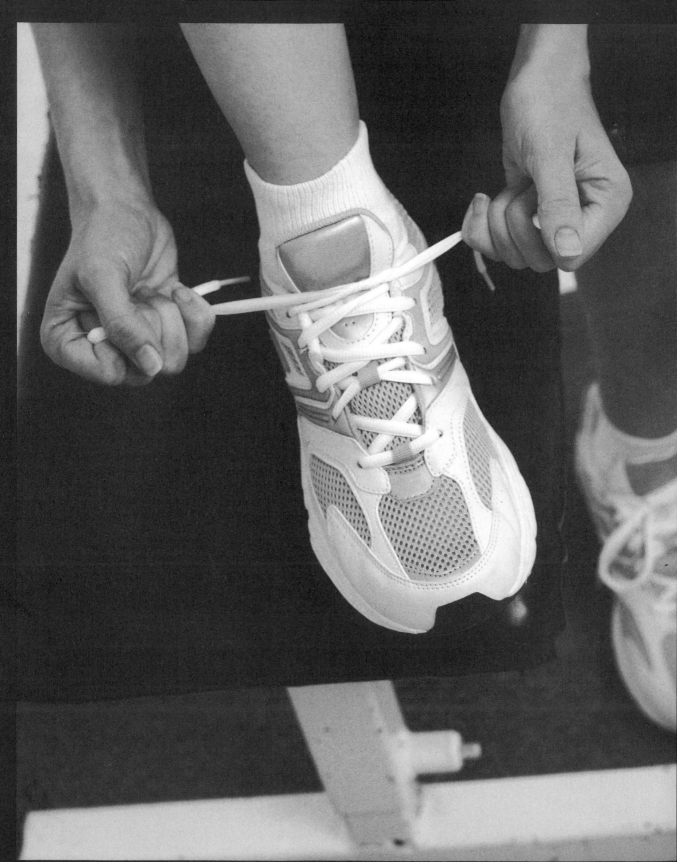

Chapter One

THE IMPLIED PREMISE AND PROMISE OF THIS BOOK ARE THAT YOU CAN CHANGE YOUR METABOLISM SO YOUR BODY IS BURNING THE OPTIMUM AMOUNT OF FAT 24 HOURS A DAY EVERY DAY OF YOUR LIFE. I WANT YOU TO KNOW FROM THE beginning that this program will not consume your life. It is designed to give you maximum results in minimal time—about three hours a week. But I will ask you to give your best during those three hours. Giving your best is another way of describing your *exercise intensity,* the level of effort you put into your workout. Rest assured, I'm not asking you to train as long and as hard as a marathon runner or Michael Jordan. They have their levels of exercise intensity, and you have yours.

All I'm asking you is to work out at *your own best individual* level of intensity, even if you have not gotten out of a chair in four months. If you're not sure what your "best" is right now, don't worry. I'll help you establish that as we get further into the actual program. Every workout and every healthy meal you choose will elevate you closer to your goals. When I started working in 2003 with the *Dr. Phil* television show and Dr. Phil's *Ultimate Weight Loss Challenge,* the 13 challengers had little or no athletic ability, and

Burning Down the Fat

> **❝** I lost 141 pounds in 9 months. Robert helped me to craft the perfect exercise routine. He continues to support me with his knowledge, guidance, trust, and friendship on my journey of weight loss. I am lucky to have learned from Robert. He practices what he teaches, and it is rare to find that honor in someone. Robert is definitely at the forefront in the field of health and exercise! **❞**
>
> ## Jim Toth
> WINNER OF DR. PHIL'S *Ultimate Weight Loss Challenge*

most were severely overweight. Yet every challenger made significant improvements over time, as much as doubling the weight he or she could lift or the speed at which he or she could walk, jog, or do other forms of cardio. It was truly amazing.

One memorable example was Jim Toth, who weighed 360 pounds when I started working with him on the *Ultimate Weight Loss Challenge*. Depressed and angry, Jim led a very negative life, even though as a popular deejay in Chicago he projected a fun-loving personality. Being overweight was part of his gig, and his audience often egged him on to eat more.

Jim had hated exercise his whole life. He ate three gargantuan meals a day, usually in his car on the way to and from work. His weight interfered with intimacy with his wife. He was ashamed of his body and ashamed of himself. He hated himself and felt like there was no escape from being overweight.

I'll never forget assessing the fitness levels of the challengers for one of the first *Dr. Phil* show tapings. They had to run or walk 100 yards as part of the assessment. Jim attacked that course like it was nobody's business. I was stunned. Here was a fit guy in a fat suit. And seeing the look in his eyes and the inspiration that came over his entire being that day affirmed for me why I had chosen health and fitness as my life's work. I'll never forget that day. I saw the athlete in Jim, if he could just get over his laziness and take responsibility for his health.

He did. Today Jim weighs 219 pounds, after losing 141 pounds in just 9 months. He works out several times a week and has changed his eating habits. He was able to throw away his fat clothes forever, filling nine giant trash bags that he gave to charity. His weight loss changed how he views himself, how he feels, and how he relates to his wife. When Jim looks at his "before" pictures, he doesn't recognize the body, only the look of unhappiness that used to be on his face.

You are fully capable of the same amount of progress. Be prepared, though: Your best will change day to day. As long as you are dedicated to the program, your best will get better!

Metabolism—The Engine of Life

This program is geared toward accelerating your metabolism so that you can burn an optimum amount of fat 24 hours a day. That's a promise I'm sure you've heard many, many times before. I'm also sure you've heard the claims of just about every diet, every weight loss plan, or every diet supplement in the drugstore that they will help you accelerate your metabolism. Many of these claims are based on phony science or are just downright unproven. With so many different theories floating about on the best way to influence your metabolism, it's hard to know what or whom to believe. This book, by contrast, is built on a sturdy scientific foundation of exercise physiology, presented here in a single, unique program that will change the way your body works and looks.

While you may think of your metabolism simply in terms of how slow or sluggish it seems to be, it is in fact nothing less than *the engine of life*. It is responsible for helping your body burn fat as well as store fat. Your metabolism also keeps your lungs breathing, your heart beating, your kidneys filtering waste, and your core body temperature on an even keel. Metabolism varies from person to person, which is why some people can eat ice cream and still maintain svelte figures while others seem to pack on pounds at the mere sight of Rocky Road. But with this program, you can change your metabolism so that it runs at peak efficiency.

What is different about my metabolism-enhancing program is that it integrates time-efficient exercise techniques, nutrition, and newly discovered lifestyle strategies into a livable, optimally designed plan. It automatically keeps your body melting fat throughout most of the day—even when you're not exercising, even when you're not breaking a sweat.

It's not just exercise that changes your metabolism for the better; it's how you exercise, how and when you eat, how much you sleep, and how you handle stress. All of these things work in sync to create a healthy metabolism and a healthy body.

That said, let me walk you through what I call "The Big Six Metabolism Dynamics"—simple principles that underpin the *Make Over Your Metabolism* program—and you'll see why it is indeed possible for you to burn fat 24-7.

The Big Six Metabolism Dynamics
Metabolism Dynamic #1: Muscle

The greatest impact on your metabolism is the amount of lean muscle you have relative to the rest of your body weight. Unlike fat, which primarily stores calories, muscle causes your body to use calories. This translates into weight loss, but more specifically into fat loss—*permanent fat loss*. Because more energy is required to maintain muscle mass, the more muscle you have, the more calories your body will burn. Having muscle is like having fireplaces lit all over your body to incinerate body fat. For every 1 pound of muscle mass you carry, you'll burn about 50 calories a day. As a result your body is burning optimum levels of body fat 24-7, even when you're sound asleep or just sitting around.

Fat tissue isn't entirely passive though. Just like the thyroid, pancreas, and adrenal glands, it secretes hormones that influence how your body works. Fat cells secrete a hormone called leptin, a naturally occurring hormone that, in normal body levels, helps regulate body fat by acting as an appetite suppressor. To a certain extent you can normalize leptin levels by increasing your level of physical activity, cutting back on saturated dietary fats (found mostly in animal fats), eliminating unhealthy fats called "trans fats" altogether, and avoiding diets that overly restrict calories.

But back to muscle. If you're among my women readers, don't let the word "muscle" scare you or make you worry that you'll put on too much of it. You won't. Unlike men, women simply don't have the hormonal makeup to build bulky mounds of muscle. The main hormone I'm talking about here is testosterone; it's the most powerful anabolic hormone in the body, meaning that it builds muscle. Men have 10 times more testosterone than women do, which is why men can generate far greater muscle growth. The muscle that women develop shows up as "definition." By that I mean a clearly visible outline of firm muscle shape that's sexy and attractive.

A good example of the remarkable results a woman can achieve through this program is Sara Kane, age 59, a psychotherapist in California. I've worked with Sara for more than five years. She had worked with several "celebrity trainers" until she was referred to me. Wanting to be fit, firm, and metabolically healthy, Sara has faithfully followed the resistance training and cardio program I developed for her—essentially the *Make Over Your Metabolism* program I put together for you in this book. She

> **"** Robert is genuinely concerned with my success. The program he created is tailor-made to meet my specific individual needs. He looks at this from a perspective of total lifestyle: exercise, nutrition, stress management, sleep, and other issues that have had an impact on my health and life during the five years that I have worked with him. I'm 59 years of age and divorced within the last two years. As a result of this lifestyle change, I wanted my program to be stepped up to the next level. And I must say it's working. Since my divorce I have not dated a guy over 40 years old! **"**
>
> ## Sara Kane
> AGE 59. CLIENT OF ROBERT REAMES

sticks to my Nutritional Life Plan. In addition she takes to heart my other metabolism-enhancing lifestyle tips. To look at Sara, you would never, ever believe she is 59. At 5 foot 2 and a firm, lean 106 pounds, she looks phenomenal.

As Sara and others with whom I've worked have discovered, the most important mode for developing lean, precious, active, valuable fat-burning muscle is resistance training (also called strength training). Resistance training involves the use of free weights (dumbbells and barbells), machines, exercise tubing, your own body weight, and other devices to challenge your muscles to work harder each time they are trained to stimulate development. My plan teaches you how to build and firm muscle in the least amount of time possible with a focused, comprehensive resistance training program designed to maximize fat burning. The exercises you'll do are designed to stimulate your major muscle groups; this activates more muscle and triggers more muscle development. The entire program centers on concise full-body exercises, specialized workouts to spot-condition your trouble areas, decreased rest between exercise sets, and a special sequence of exercising that includes some cardio along with your favorite

> **"** I had the opportunity to work with Robert during Dr. Phil's *Ultimate Weight Loss Challenge*. He developed my exercise program, which consisted of strength training and cardiovascular exercises. He guided me as to when and how much to increase my intensity levels to receive the full benefit of my workouts. Robert is patient and thorough. His support has helped to make me the person I am today. I never thought I would say this, but I love exercising! I love my new look and I love the transformation that my body has taken on. When you look up the word 'angel,' Robert's name should be beside it because he was definitely God sent. To date I have lost 85 pounds! **"**
>
> ## Judith Blowe
> PARTICIPANT ON DR. PHIL'S *Ultimate Weight Loss Challenge*

sports/recreational activities. When used together these techniques increase the fat-burning potential of your body's muscles.

A critical aspect of the resistance training you'll do on this program is that it is high-intensity, meaning that you push as hard as you can in your workouts but without spending a great deal of time doing so—no more than 30 minutes three times a week. High-intensity resistance training is a bona fide way to lose body fat and control your weight—not only because it develops calorie-burning muscle, but also because it boosts your body's ability to keep burning calories for many hours after you train. In a study done at Ohio University, volunteers performed a high-intensity resistance training workout that lasted just 30 minutes. The exercisers pushed each exercise to "failure," the point at which they could not do another repetition, no matter how hard they tried. The study's objective was to learn how long calorie burning would last beyond the initial workout. By measuring oxygen consumption (a marker of calorie burning), the researchers discovered that the exercisers were still burning additional calories for up to 38 hours after they had worked out! This effect is what I call metabolic afterburn, and I explain it in detail below. Not coincidentally, this is exactly the same type of workout you'll do on my plan—a high-intensity, 30-minute, full-body resistance training routine. It is an important part of the strategy to turn your body into a fat-burning, calorie-burning machine 24-7.

What about cardio, or aerobic, exercise? Because cardio strengthens your heart and lungs and is an effective component of a fat-loss strategy, I am very much in favor of it. But as I caution my clients, be careful about overdoing cardio. Why? Excess cardio can curtail levels of important hormones. In other words if you go overboard trying to burn calories with cardio, you may lower hormone levels that help burn fat and build muscle. What's more, you may lose muscle mass. The result is that you can end up looking soft and not at all firm.

There's more to the hormone story. Too much cardio can cause your body to churn out excesses of a hormone called cortisol. Cortisol is released when your body faces any type of stress, including too much exercise. When cortisol is elevated your body can begin to prioritize muscle tissue as an energy source, tearing it down instead of building it up. Losing muscle tissue can cause your metabolism to slow down. You'll hear a lot about cortisol in this book, and how to control it, because it has so many other implications in metabolism and weight gain.

Excessive cardio can exhaust your adrenal glands too, leading to fatigue. Often called the "glands of stress," the adrenal glands help your body deal with stress from every angle, ranging from injury and disease to job and relationship problems. Your energy and ability to bounce back from stress depend on the proper functioning of these glands.

You will find out that just three 30-minute sessions of a type of cardio called Metabolic Burst Training is the max you need to do to keep your hormonal levels stable, your metabolism on the ascent, and your body fat on the decline. I discuss Metabolic Burst Training options on pages 21, 91 and in Chapters 6 and 7.

As beneficial as cardio is, alone it is not enough to upgrade your metabolism. You also must develop and reshape your muscles with resistance training. Only by working with resistance can you transform soft and flabby body parts into tight, firm muscles—and get a supercharged metabolism in the process.

Metabolism Dynamic #2: Afterburn

If you're like most people, you probably love the idea of getting a big return on your investment. So I'll bet you're probably going to love the idea of metabolic afterburn, or as it is technically known, "excess postexercise oxygen consumption" (EPOC) or "oxygen debt." Metabolic afterburn refers to the extra calories you burn once your workout is over and you've headed for the shower and are ready to carry on your day.

When you exercise you burn calories during the workout to fuel your muscles. In 1 hour of working out, for example, you can burn roughly 350 to 500 calories. That's great, though not a huge amount because you need to burn about 3,500 calories to shed 1 pound of body fat. The number of calories you burn during your workout is certainly important, and they all add up, but these calories aren't quite as critical to your metabolism as how many you burn after your workout. After being exercised your body keeps on burning even more calories from glucose and fat. This caloric dividend, paid after the investment of exercising, is the essence of metabolic afterburn.

But do you know why it happens, or better yet, the best way to maximize this effect?

At a physiological level, your body continues to require and use oxygen at a higher rate than before the exercise began in order to repay the oxygen debt. Oxygen is what your body employs to restore itself to a resting state. When oxygen is consumed at an elevated rate, energy is also being consumed at an elevated rate. Since oxygen is used to burn calories, your body heads into this calorie-burning zone and stays there for up to 24 hours, and sometimes up to 48 hours, after you have worked out.

Several different mechanisms explain why afterburn occurs as your body returns to its pre-exercise state. Your body continues to expend energy after exercise to re-oxygenate your blood, for example, and restore circulatory hormones. Energy molecules must be regenerated, along with muscle glycogen (a stored form of glucose) that was used for fuel during exercise. Oxygen is required to help remove and reuse the lactic acid your muscles have created. As energy is released from exercising muscles, heat is produced. This necessitates energy expenditure after exercise to return your body to its normal core temperature. In addition your body uses up energy to return your breathing and your heart rate to normal. Most of these processes are fueled by body fat and are the underlying reasons why your metabolism keeps ticking after exercise.

How long the calorie burning continues depends on numerous factors, including the type of exercise and its intensity, meaning you can use this science to make your workouts as effective as possible. Here are the ways in which you will maximize your own metabolic afterburn while following this program:

- **Follow a consistent routine** of resistance training in order to stimulate the development of calorie-burning muscle. Like the study I cited on page 18, much research shows that resistance training produces a greater afterburn than aerobic exercise does. The reason? More energy is required to restore bodily systems to normal.

- **Give your personal best level of intensity** during every exercise session. The more intense your resistance training workouts, the greater the metabolic afterburn, studies show.

- **Try to keep your rest periods** between exercise sets as brief as possible—30 to 45 seconds to as much as one minute, on average. Shorter rest periods stimulate higher production of lactic acid and thus increase the need for oxygen to remove it.

- **Employ multiple sets** (two, three, or up to as many as eight sets per body part) in order to stimulate hormonal changes and metabolic demands.

- **Incorporate as much variety** into your workouts as possible because your body loves the element of change. What's more, variety promotes muscular development.

- **Carefully follow my program** of Metabolic Burst Training (see below), an exercise system that stimulates an even greater metabolic afterburn.

As you will soon discover, the workouts in this program are optimally designed, taking advantage of all of the above factors, so you can maximize your metabolic afterburn, continue to burn calories for up to 48 hours after your exercise session, and launch a successful attack on your body's fat stores. For the three hours a week you'll put in, that's a terrific investment. Wouldn't you agree?

Metabolism Dynamic #3: Metabolic Burst Training

As a personal trainer, consultant, and nutritionist to many clients who have busy lives, it is my job to produce results for them in as little time as possible. One of the methods I use and strongly endorse is Metabolic Burst Training (also known as interval training). Metabolic Burst Training is simply alternating short higher-intensity spurts of increased cardio activity with spurts of less-intense cardio activity in your workout. Let's use walking, for example, either outdoors or on a treadmill. After properly warming up, you'd jog for one minute, then walk for one minute. Or you could do one-minute sprints interspersed with one-minute jogs. The beauty of Metabolic Burst Training is that you can do it for any aerobic activity you perform, from cycling and swimming to exercising on cardio machines. The benefits of Metabolic Burst Training are terrific—and verified by a huge body of research. The benefits include the following:

21

Maximizes your afterburn. Metabolic Burst Training offers the bonus of further stimulating the afterburn described earlier. After higher-intensity exercise, your body requires extra energy to repair muscles, re-tank energy stores, repay the "oxygen debt," and basically restore your body to its normal state. These recovery processes can take up to a full day, which is why you continue to burn calories and fat for hours after your workout. In fact research shows that if you do interval training just twice a week, you can lose twice as much weight as someone who does just a regular moderate cardio workout, probably due to this positive metabolic effect.

Favors fat burning. I realize that one of the biggest reasons you've purchased this book is because you want to rid your body of unsightly fat. I have great news for you: Metabolic Burst Training favors the use of fat for fuel and taps into fat stores more efficiently than conventional aerobic exercise. Researchers have actually biopsied the muscle tissue of exercisers before and after various training programs. They found that Metabolic Burst Training increases the activity of fat-burning enzymes in muscles to a greater extent than other forms of lower- or moderate-intensity aerobic training. What's more they've discovered that only during burst-type training does fat that is located within the muscle break down into particles called fatty acids, which provide the actual fuel burned for exercise. Put simply, Metabolic Burst Training is a pure fat burner!

Increases human growth hormone. During higher-intensity bursts of effort, your body secretes hormones. Among the more beneficial of these hormones is human growth hormone, which mobilizes fat for fuel by increasing its presence in your bloodstream. It also encourages your body to synthesize muscle-forming protein. Blood levels of this hormone rise significantly during and immediately after higher-intensity Metabolic Burst Training, whereas levels rise very little or remain the same during and after low- or moderate-intensity aerobic exercise.

Builds variety into your workout. Variety is a surefire way to prevent boredom from setting in so that you can continue to lose weight. If your workouts are less monotonous and more fun, you're more apt to stick to exercising as a matter of habit. Doing so will get you in shape and keep you there, plus increase your fitness. With Metabolic Burst Training you can always change your routine and try different activities. This is important because your body adapts after about four weeks of doing the same activity and becomes less efficient at burning fat.

Builds cardiovascular fitness. Like conventional aerobic exercise, Metabolic Burst Training also promotes the fitness of your heart and lungs. However, the higher intensity of Burst Training demands more oxygen for your working muscles. Consequently,

> **"**As a family, we lost 234 pounds. Without the help of Robert leading the way for our fitness plan it will never be known if we could have become the winners of the *Ultimate Family Weight Loss Challenge*. One thing is thoroughly clear to us today. You can have a trainer, but with Robert Reames we were led by the best of the best, and he took us to the finish line. Thank you, Robert, for your expertise and helping us to achieve our family's victorious win and magnificent weight loss. And thank you for an education in health and exercise that will keep us in shape for the rest of our lives!**"**
>
> ## Vic, Pennie, Luke, and Jake Pennington
> WINNERS, DR. PHIL'S *Ultimate Family Weight Loss Challenge*

your heart adapts by raising both heart rate and stroke volume (the amount of blood pumped out per heartbeat) to provide oxygenated blood. This increased pumping power makes your heart stronger and more efficient. Plus every heartbeat delivers more blood at rest as well as during exercise. There's more: Burst Training has been found in research to increase levels of high-density lipoprotein cholesterol (HDL)—that's the good kind that is partly responsible for keeping your arteries healthy and free from clogging. Bottom line: There are several chief cardiovascular benefits of Metabolic Burst Training.

Metabolism Dynamic #4: Nutrition

Anyone who has ever tried to wash dishes in water without dish soap knows it just isn't going to work. Likewise, you're not going to burn an optimal amount of fat without exercise *and* the right nutrition plan. You need both. My Nutritional Life Plan provides the correct balance of protein, carbohydrates, and fat to help accelerate your metabolism; teaches you how to time your carb intake for maximum benefit; and focuses on the number of meals and snacks eaten daily. It's a practical, easy approach to nutrition that makes losing weight easier and puts you in control of your meals.

With my Nutritional Life Plan you'll get plenty of protein, and this will boost your metabolism, causing you to burn an extra 150 to 200 calories a day. That's because protein is composed of amino acids, which are harder for your body to break down, causing you to burn more calories. Protein at each meal also significantly helps you avoid cravings by helping to balance your blood sugar levels.

I hope you'll be relieved when I tell you that my Nutritional Life Plan is not low-carb. Instead it includes good carbohydrates that have a healthy effect on your metabolism. You see, poor nutritional habits such as eating processed carbohydrates and sweets increase the levels of insulin in your body. Insulin is an important hormone, one that is produced in the pancreas. Most of its actions are directed at the metabolism of carbohydrates, fats, and proteins. It works by ushering glucose into cells to be burned for energy. Many people in this country are insulin resistant. This is a condition in which the body doesn't respond as well to the insulin that the pancreas is making, and glucose is less able to enter the cells. Consequently, higher levels of insulin are required in order for insulin to do its job. Unfortunately, elevated insulin can prompt your body to store more fat and actually slow your metabolism. This interplay between food, insulin activity, and insulin resistance is one of the major reasons people in the United States have so much trouble losing weight. Among other benefits, my Nutritional Life Plan helps to *increase* your body's *sensitivity* to insulin.

You'll also eat throughout the day to lose body fat. Eating to lose fat sounds counter-intuitive, but it works. Eating five to six smaller meals a day as opposed to three squares keeps your metabolism going 24-7 too.

Let's face it: Americans are obsessed with food. I want to keep us obsessed with food—delicious, healthy, good-for-you food that you can eat five times a day and still lose weight. I'm talking about real food as opposed to fake and overly processed food. That stuff is foreign to our systems; our bodies just downright don't know what to do with it. My Nutritional Life Plan hones in on real foods, which truly is what we need to be eating for a healthy metabolism. I also want you to change your thinking about food. Clean your cabinets, refrigerators, and freezers *now* to get rid of foods that do not support your healthy goals.

Metabolism Dynamic #5: Sleep

The fact that you've had trouble losing weight isn't solely from your pizza, ice cream, or potato chip habit. It may stem from not getting enough sleep. Sleep deprivation is a leading factor in weight gain. It may make you put on pounds by disrupting hormones (insulin, cortisol, ghrelin, leptin, growth hormone, and thyroid hormones) that control your eating habits and metabolism, seriously sabotaging your weight loss efforts. Plus, when you're tired your body doesn't have the energy to do its normal day-to-day functions—including burning calories—so your metabolism slows to a crawl.

It may not be a coincidence that the prevalence of obesity has been increasing over the recent decades—in parallel with the rise in insomnia. This relationship between obesity and sleep deprivation has prompted a flurry of research studies. In one study conducted at Eastern Virginia Medical School in Virginia, 924 volunteers between the ages of 18 and 91 were put into four groups according to weight (normal weight, over-weight, obese, and extremely obese). They filled out questionnaires about their demographics, medical habits, sleep habits, and use of substances such as caffeine, tobacco, alcohol, and weight-loss products that could affect the quality of their sleep.

The Virginia researchers found that the normal-weight volunteers slept, on average, 16 minutes longer each night than those in the other groups. That may not seem like a huge amount, but over a week's time it adds up to almost two hours of sleep. Their conclusion: "Reduced amounts of sleep are associated with overweight and obese status."

There is a wealth of other studies that draw similar conclusions, which all goes to show: One of the best lifestyle patterns you can weave into your life for weight loss and control is to get a full night's sleep. It will keep your metabolic energy running high, stabilize hormonal levels, contribute to the development of calorie-burning muscle, and even reduce carbohydrate cravings. And curbing cravings is a key component to my Nutritional Life Plan. In Chapter 2 we will talk about the lifestyle issue of sleep in detail and how getting more of it may just help you weigh less.

Metabolism Dynamic #6: Stress

Another cause of extra weight, particularly around your middle, may be stress. When you feel eternally stressed out, your body is flooded with stress hormones such as cortisol. If stress goes unresolved, these hormones trigger fat cells in the abdomen to increase in size and encourage fat storage. Cortisol automatically kicks up your appetite, prompting a ravenous urge to eat everything in sight, especially sweets and refined carbohydrates (foods that make insulin levels soar, then collapse, leaving you feeling hungrier than ever). You end up eating many more calories than you can burn off.

No matter how healthy your diet is, chronically high levels of cortisol can make you pack on pounds. So it is absolutely critical that you get a grip on the stress in your life. The stress-management tools you will learn in Chapter 2 will help you melt away pounds, particularly when used in partnership with exercise and nutritious eating.

Why This Program Will Work for You

Based on these six dynamics, the *Make Over Your Metabolism* program will help you manage your weight, shape, and appetite by providing a time-efficient, fat-burning exercise plan, a supersimple nutrition plan that will optimize your metabolism, and lifestyle strategies that will help correct red flags that interfere with a healthy metabolism.

This is not a temporary program that will leave you stranded at the end. This is a plan and a continuous source of reference that can stay with you for life. No matter what your present level of physical ability is, no matter what condition you're in, no matter what you've done in the past, you have the ability to achieve success on this program and become the fittest and very best version of yourself. Everyone wins on this plan.

Hormones and Your Metabolism

One of the most important elements of losing body fat is the level of your hormones. Hormones are chemicals that your body manufactures naturally and releases into your bloodstream, and their levels can make or break your weight-control efforts. The *Make Over Your Metabolism* program is designed to help optimize levels of key hormones, and I'll be talking about them throughout this book. This chart defines all sorts of hormones involved in fat burning and muscle development and summarizes how they can be controlled with the diet, exercise, and lifestyle strategies you'll apply on this program.

Hormone	What It Does	How to Control It
Cortisol	Facilitates fat retention, particularly in the abdominal area.	Get adequate sleep. (People suffering from sleep deprivation tend to have higher levels of cortisol.) Reduce stress levels by relaxing more and incorporating stress-reduction techniques.

Hormones and Your Metabolism

Hormone	What It Does	How to Control It
Ghrelin	Boosts your appetite and signals your body to keep eating.	Avoid getting really hungry; eat several healthy meals throughout the day. Increase your daily intake of fiber. Get adequate sleep. (People suffering from sleep deprivation tend to have higher levels of ghrelin.)
Glucagon	Keeps blood sugar even and unlocks fat stores for energy usage.	Include adequate protein in your diet. Eating protein causes your body to release glucagon.
Growth Hormone	Promotes the development of lean muscle mass and the reduction of body fat. Has significantly positive effects against premature aging.	Follow a program of resistance training that incorporates moderately heavy resistance with no more than one minute of rest between sets. Include Metabolic Burst Training as part of your fat-loss efforts.
Insulin	Ushers glucose into cells for energy; can be a fat-forming hormone when overly elevated or when cells become insensitive to insulin.	Avoid processed carbohydrates and sugary foods. Maintain a regular program of resistance training, cardio training, and overall physical activity. Keep your weight under control.
Leptin	Helps your body regulate its weight.	Decrease dietary fat. Increase physical activity. Avoid restrictive dieting or fasting.
Thyroid Hormones	Help to curb appetite. Regulate how many calories your body burns each day. Influence muscle development by speeding up or slowing down protein synthesis. Greatly affect the regulation of your overall metabolism.	Avoid restrictive dieting, which causes thyroid hormone levels to fall, generating a negative effect on metabolism. Consult with your physician regarding optimum thyroid treatment for you.

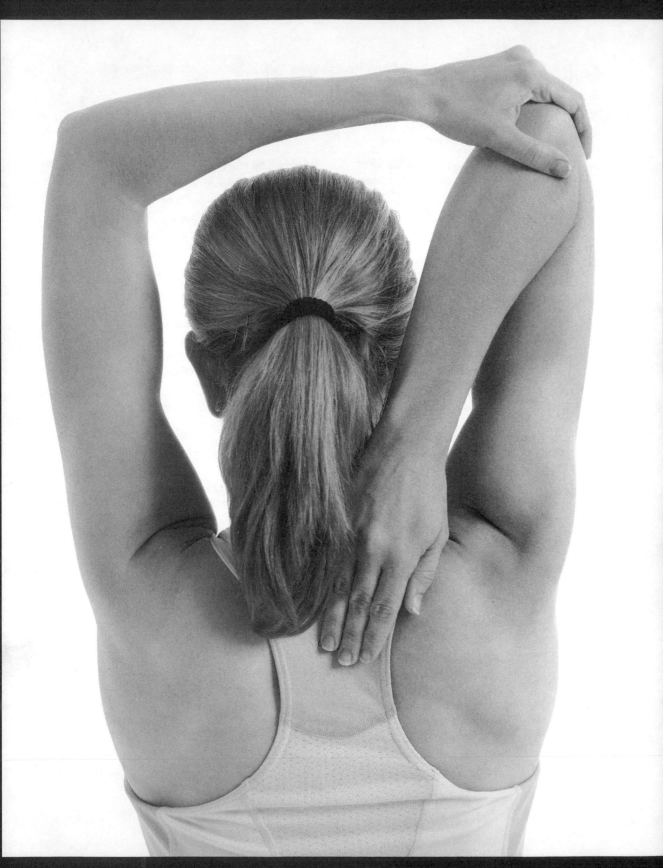

Chapter Two

WHEN YOU THINK ABOUT BURNING FAT AND INCREASING YOUR METABO-
LISM, THE FIRST METHOD THAT COMES TO MIND IS EXERCISE. YES, THAT'S
A TRIED-AND-TRUE WAY TO DO IT AND A MAJOR COMPONENT OF THIS
program, but there is much more that is involved. If I told you that sleep and stress management are intricately involved in metabolic health, I bet you'd think I was crazy. But
I'm not! Truth be told, there is a huge body of research proving that metabolism is
strongly affected, in good ways and bad, by how much sleep you get, the quality of that
sleep, and how well you contend with the stress in your life.

The *Make Over Your Metabolism* program is a total lifestyle approach to weight loss,
fat loss, and metabolic health; exercising and eating right are key components, but
they don't work in isolation. As we go through this program together, I want you to
take a long, hard look at your sleep and stress-management habits and, if necessary,
improve them. I'll give you some easy-to-follow strategies. Remember, we are
revamping your metabolism so that you burn fat at *your* optimum level 24-7, and you
need all your "metabolic ducks" in a row to make this happen. You must get adequate

Metabolism Maximizers

sleep and be able to minimize and cope with stress, or you're only partway to achieving your metabolic goals. I want you to do everything within your power to get in the greatest shape of your life.

Metabolism and Stress

The prevailing notion is that poor diet and lack of exercise are the main causes of unsightly fat on our bodies, and that is absolutely true. But one little-known culprit in unsuccessful weight control is stress. Emotional or mental tension accelerates our heart rate, elevates our blood pressure, tenses our muscles, and places us in "fight or flight" mode. Too much of the wrong kind of stress, or chronic stress, inflicts damage on our physical, emotional, and spiritual well-being.

Stress is something that we realistically cannot escape. To be alive is to be under a certain amount of stress. Although you cannot always control the external situations that bring on stress, you can control your reaction to them using a variety of strategies that I'll describe in this section.

Stress is related intricately to overall health. Your body churns out hormones in response to stress in your life. Over time, these hormones may wind up contributing to heart disease, high blood pressure, suppressed immunity, digestive problems, and even depression. One of the hormones, cortisol, is so detrimental to weight control that it will drive you straight to your favorite fattening, sugary comfort foods to replenish the energy your body used up in coping with a stressful situation. As a result, you can end up eating more calories than you can burn off.

When you're chronically stressed out, your body keeps releasing cortisol, so you're even more prone to overeating the wrong foods. Cortisol tells your body to store fat, particularly in your midsection. As fat cells there increase, so does your risk of heart disease, diabetes, and certain cancers.

Be encouraged, though, that you can overcome stress-induced weight gain by making some very simple changes that involve diet, exercise, and important stress-management tools. As we go over these, I think you'll find that this aspect of weight management is totally within your control. You'll feel relieved that you have the power not only to manage your weight but also to gain the upper hand on stress in your life. You'll be happier, more at peace, and infinitely more in charge of your life. And that is a wonderful gift to give yourself. Stress is an enemy to metabolic control. And you'll benefit greatly from these strategies to manage it. Here are some steps you can begin to take today and as we progress through this program.

- **Free yourself from dieting obsessions.** When you obsess over your food choices, whether by counting calories, fat, or carbs, you create stress in your life. Research shows that women who obsess over what they eat produce more cortisol than those who are not fixated on food. Eating should never be a stressful experience. Food is fuel and nutrition for your body. Try to focus on the true nature of food—it's a substance that exists to keep you healthy and help your body perform at its optimal capacity. I'm encouraging you to change your "food attitude," seeing food less as a form of entertainment and more as sustenance for life.

- **Choose the right foods.** You'll learn more about healthy food choices in my Nutritional Life Plan, covered in Chapters 8 and 9. But for now let me recommend that you rid your home of junk food such as cookies, commercially baked foods, high-sugar cereals, candy, and sweets. These foods—considered "refined carbohydrates"—trigger a reaction in your body that leads to the release of more fat-forming cortisol. Not only that, these foods also wreak havoc with your insulin levels, setting off food cravings as your blood sugar seesaws. Ridding your diet of refined carbs will help greatly to stabilize and balance your insulin and blood sugar levels.

  There isn't a food you can eat that will tame cortisol, but it is clearly much better for your metabolic health to choose natural, unprocessed foods such as fruits, vegetables, and whole grains as the centerpiece of your diet to prevent weight-gain-triggering hormonal responses.

  Protein choices are important too. Try to eat at least three or four servings of fish a week, as my Nutritional Life Plan suggests. Fish such as tuna and salmon are high in omega-3 fatty acids, which help control mood so you're less likely to engage in stress eating. Also, protein combined with healthy fats—which I call "thin fats"—helps keep your metabolism high.

- **Bypass stress when you can.** You know what the stressors are in your life. Traffic, deadlines, being overscheduled and overcommitted, certain people, poor nutrition, financial problems, work demands, negative self-talk, perfectionism—to name just a few. If you feel overwhelmed, pay more attention to what stresses you out and avoid the stress-inducing situations. For instance if you're always rushing and hurrying from one activity to another and never catching up, you may need to work on time management and organization.

- **Keep a realistic perspective.** Think about this for a moment: Do you get stressed out thinking about things that are out of your control or events that aren't going to happen for a long time? To become less stress-prone, take a serious look at what you can control and what you cannot. For example if your family life feels chaotic because you're shuttling your kids to soccer practice, ballet, language lessons, and everywhere in between, you have control over that schedule. You can cut back on some activities to rebalance your life and reduce the chaos. There is a familiar prayer that speaks thoughtfully to this issue: "God, grant me the serenity to accept the things I cannot change; courage to change the things I can; and the wisdom to know the difference."

  Also stay focused on today and don't worry about something coming up in the future, because it may or may not happen. If you stress out about all the problems now and possible ones in the future, you're going to feel like you're going over the edge. Remind yourself: Everything works out in the end.

- **Talk it out.** Stress is often caused by a skewed perception of reality. We get caught up in a problem, take a negative view of something that's going on, or turn a minor situation into a catastrophe. In these situations it is therapeutic to discuss your problems with a trusted friend, someone from your house of worship, or a counselor. Doing so can give you a more accurate, rational perspective on events, reducing stress and giving you a sense of control over your life.

- **Clarify your life goals.** Many times feelings of stress are caused by a sense of hopelessness or loss of aim in life. We may make choices that won't fulfill us. You might be in a job that feels like a dead end, when you would be better suited to another profession. If this describes you, decide what you really want out of your life. The more fulfilled you feel with your career and your personal life, the better you can cope with the day-to-day stresses. It is important to take control over your destiny without sacrificing the well-being of your family. By doing so you can lead a life that challenges and uplifts you.

- **Keep moving.** It is no big secret that exercising is one of the best ways to relieve stress. Every time you work out, your body releases endorphins—feel-good chemicals that boost your mood, block pain, help you relax, and keep stress hormones like cortisol in check.

Of course there are peripheral benefits to exercising as well. The self-confidence that comes with weight loss and improved body image positively affects your overall outlook on life and your mood.

Performing the exercise routines I've outlined in this book, including the De-Stress Stretch program below, will reduce stress hormones and make you much more resilient to stress in your life.

Robert's De-Stress Stretch Program

When you're feeling tense and stressed out, the De-Stress Stretch program on the following pages will bring you near-instant calm. Physiologically, stretching blunts the stress hormone response, increases circulation of blood and oxygen to your muscles, releases tension, and improves flexibility. Relax your body when performing this stretch routine. Just as I encourage your highest level of intensity during aerobic and stretch training workouts, for your De-Stress Stretch I encourage the ultimate in relaxation and calm. Breathe into these stretches, relax, clear your mind, put on some of your favorite calming music or listen to the sounds of silence, and enjoy. If you incorporate this program into your life, using it on days when you feel overwhelmed, you'll take back your power over stress and feel so much better for it. Please refer to "Robert's Rules to Stretch By" below and on page 150. For more information on stability balls, including what size to buy, see page 77.

ROBERT'S RULES TO STRETCH BY

•Stretching motions should be gradual and gentle, not fast or jerky. •Hold each stretch in a static position for 10–15 seconds. •Never "bounce" during stretches. •Stretch only to the point of comfortably "feeling it." If the stretch is painful, you've gone too far. •Take your time with your stretching routine. Stretching will help your body recover, both physically and mentally.

1. STANDING LIFT AND BREATHE

Target: whole-body relaxation

Positioning: Stand nice and tall with your feet firmly planted on the floor and your knees slightly bent. Begin with your arms crossed in front of you.

Motion: Inhale while lifting your arms to the sky and exhale as you return to the original position. Perform this stretch twice.

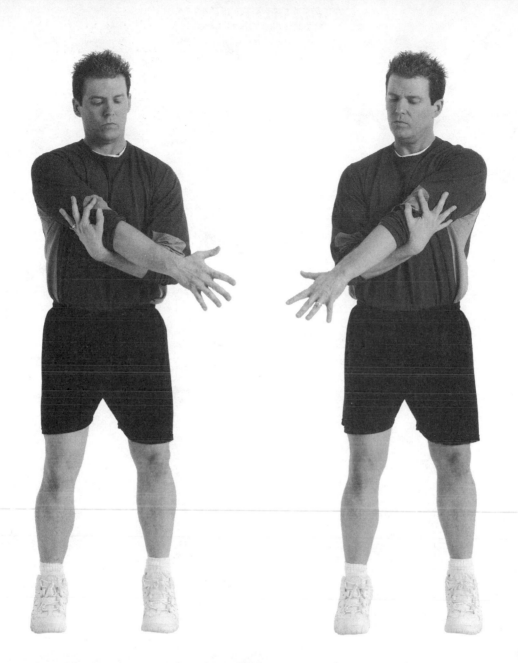

2. STANDING SHOULDER STRETCH

Target: entire shoulder area, with rear shoulder focus

Positioning: Stand nice and tall with your feet firmly planted on the floor and your knees slightly bent. Activate your supercenter (see page 89 for details).

Motion: Reach your arm diagonally across your upper body, as shown, and hold for 10–15 seconds. Relax and breathe deeply into the stretch. Repeat with the other arm. Perform this stretch twice on each side.

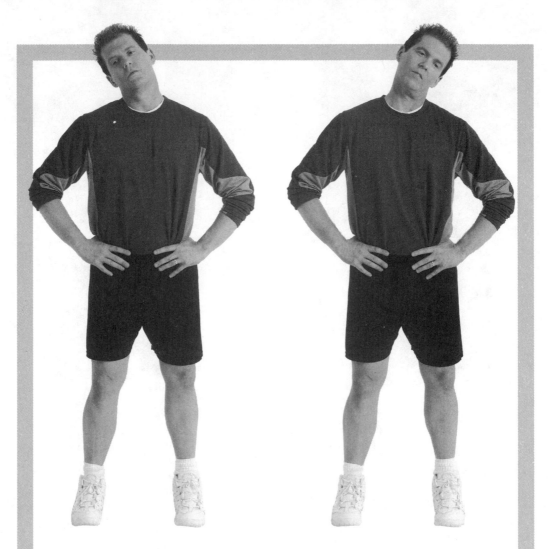

3. NECK STRETCH

Target: side of neck area

Positioning: Stand nice and tall with your feet firmly planted on the floor and your knees slightly bent. Keep your shoulders down and your neck long.

Motion: Let your head fall to your right side. Relax and breathe into the stretch. Hold for 10–15 seconds and repeat to the left side. Perform this stretch twice on each side. Keep your eyes open as you stretch! Vision is a major and necessary component of balance, stability, and overall safety.

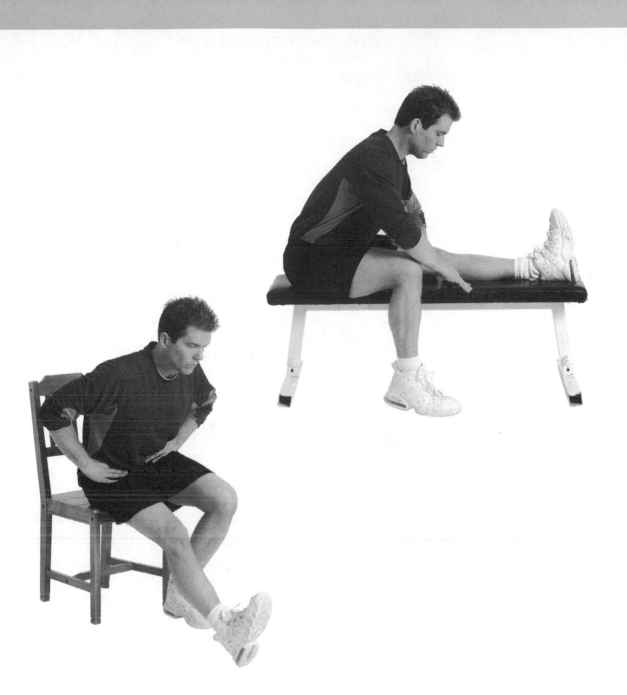

4. SEATED HAMSTRING STRETCH

Target: hamstrings, behind the knee, calf area, and low back

Positioning: Sit on a chair or bench with your back flat and outstretch one leg. Bend the other leg, placing it firmly on the floor.

Motion: Lean forward toward your outstretched leg. Relax and breathe into the stretch, holding for 10–15 seconds. Repeat the stretch on the opposite side. Perform this stretch twice on each side.

37

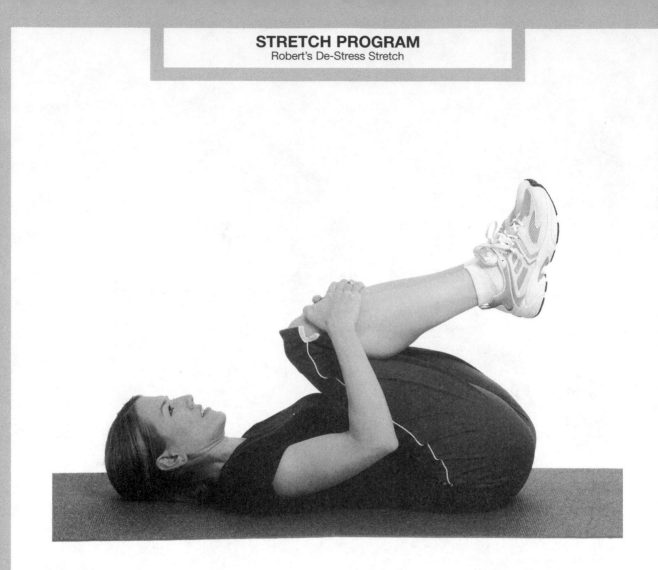

5. KNEES TO CHEST STRETCH

Target: low back and hips

Positioning: Lie faceup on the floor. Keep your head on the floor.

Motion: Bring both knees toward your chest and hold. Breathe into the stretch and hold for 10–15 seconds. Perform this stretch twice.

6. CROSSOVER HIP STRETCH

Target: glutes and total hip area

Positioning: Lie flat on your back.

Motion: Cross your right leg over your left leg and bring your left knee in toward your chest. Hold the leg in this position with your hands while keeping the back of your head on the floor. Hold the stretch for 10–15 seconds, breathing into the stretch. Repeat on the opposite side. Perform this stretch twice on each side.

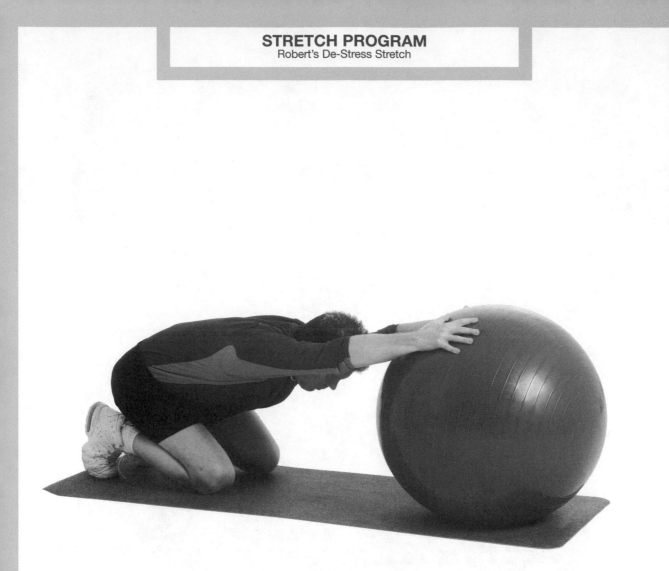

7. CHILD'S POSE

Target: comprehensive back and shoulders

Positioning: Sit in a kneeling position with your glutes toward or against the backs of your feet. Outstretch your arms on a stability ball, as shown.

Motion: Lengthen your arms while simultaneously relaxing your shoulders and back. Breathe into the stretch and repeat for a second time. Keep your eyes open!

8. SIDE-LYING BALL STRETCH

Target: lats, entire side of your body, and an area called the IT band (a layer of connective tissue that runs down the outside of your leg from the outer hip to below the knee)

Positioning: Lie sideways on the ball with your bottom leg bent to stabilize your body. Fully extend your top leg, as shown, and extend your arm overhead.

Motion: Allow your body to drape over the ball. Stretch the entire side of your body. Relax and breathe into the stretch. Hold the stretch for 10–15 seconds and repeat on the opposite side. Stretch both sides of your body twice. Keep your eyes open!

41

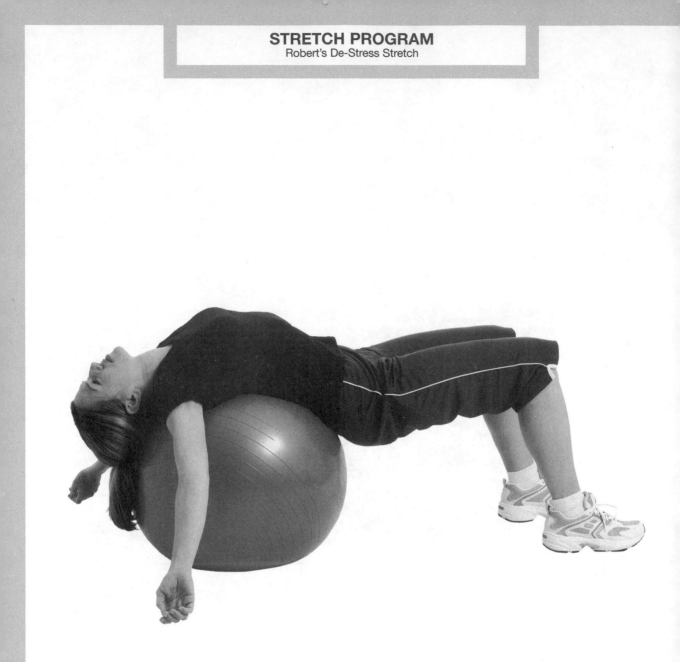

9. BALL FACEUP BACK STRETCH

Target: total back, chest, and shoulders

Positioning: Lie faceup on a stability ball. Place the ball at your mid to low back. Keep your feet planted firmly on the floor.

Motion: Allow your body to drape over the ball. Open your arms out to the side and relax your head, neck, shoulders, arms, chest, and facial muscles. Relax and breathe into the stretch. Hold for 10–15 seconds and repeat for a second time. Keep your eyes open!

10. BALL HIP FLEXOR STRETCH

Target: hip flexor area and quadriceps

Positioning: Lean forward on your bent right leg while extending your left leg back. Hold on to the ball for stability, as shown.

Motion: Keep your chest high and lean your body forward. You will feel this in the front portion of your left hip. Breathe into the stretch and hold this position for 10–15 seconds. Perform the stretch twice and repeat on the opposite side.

11. FLOOR "V" CENTER STRETCH

Target: inner thighs, hamstrings, and low back

Positioning: Sit up nice and tall, keeping your back straight. Open your legs as wide as possible.

Motion: Flex your feet, bringing your toes toward your knees, as shown. Breathe into the stretch and hold for 10–15 seconds, then repeat for a second time.

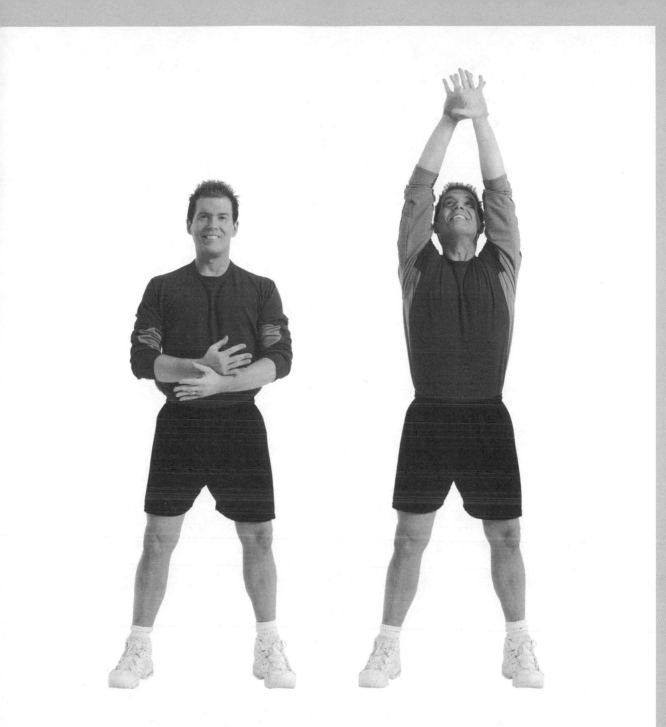

12. STANDING LIFT AND BREATHE
Repeat stretch #1 to conclude the routine. See the directions on page 34 for this exercise.

Self-Massage for Metabolic Control: You're Hearing It Here First!

Using a simple instrument called The Stick, you can give your body a massage that reduces stress hormones known to increase the accumulation of body fat, releases tension, increases strength, and makes you more limber. (For more information on purchasing and using The Stick, visit www.robertreames.net or the manufacturer's website at www.thestick.net.) This form of "self-massage" also accelerates recovery time after workouts. It increases blood flow to muscles, which is important because the blood delivers recovery nutrients to the tissues. The net effect is improved muscular development in the wake of exercising, and this, of course, enhances metabolism. For optimizing performance, relieving stress, and treating muscle discomfort, the self-massage is nearly miraculous in its results.

A case in point is Michael and his wife, Margo, who are longtime clients of mine. Michael goes all out when it comes to exercise. He takes intense power walks practically every day. But at age 63 he started developing painful tension in the top portion of his hamstring up toward his glute muscle on his left side. This condition became so unbearable that he wasn't able to do his power walks at all, and this forced layoff really concerned him. Michael's doctor advised him to do some stretching exercises, which he did, and these helped temporarily. But as he resumed his high-intensity workouts, the problem reared its painful head again.

At around that time I had begun using The Stick myself and recommending it to a few clients. I showed Michael how to use it. When we met for our training session, I had him roll The Stick over his hamstring muscles. The next day he power-walked his normal, vigorous course. Michael reported back to me that his hamstring issue had been alleviated by 70 percent—and that was after just one massage with The Stick! The next time he used it, the problem improved by another 10 percent, and Michael was convinced of the benefits of using The Stick on a regular basis. It has been more than a year now, and he has absolutely no pain or tension in that hamstring/glute area, nor does he feel the postworkout tension in his quadriceps that he had been experiencing. I showed Margo how to use The Stick too, and the results have been fantastic in improving her posture and relieving her neck and back discomfort. Before using The Stick and incorporating my "supercenter" work (which you will see in Chapter 6), she had been subject to habitual shoulder, back, and neck tension, with her shoulders stooped forward. Self-massage work has proved invaluable for relief, comfort, balance, and optimum postural alignment. As a result she's made incredible gains in her overall strength and stamina both in her exercise program and in activities of daily living.

One of the pluses of The Stick is that you can use it on your own—no need to pay expensive massage fees. (However, I do *highly* recommend a periodic massage from a certified or licensed practitioner. Research shows that this greatly enhances your overall health and ability to control your weight.)

All it takes is two to five minutes of self-massage on the body parts you want to work. You can do this anytime, including after a workout, to restore flexibility and

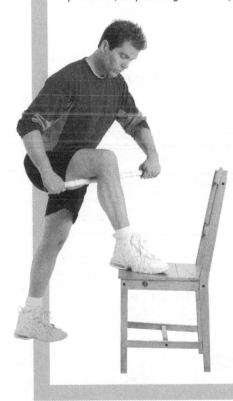

To perform self-massage, simply grasp The Stick on both sides and begin rolling it over a body part as if you were rolling out a piecrust. You can apply more or less pressure, depending on how you feel. Some other important guidelines:

• Keep your muscles relaxed while using The Stick.
• Use The Stick directly on your skin or through light clothing.
• For best results, use The Stick before, during, and after periods of activity.
• Avoid excessive use, as this may cause muscle soreness. The Stick comes with basic instructions on how to perform your own self-massage.
• A typical full-body self-massage would be as follows: low back, 25–30 seconds; hamstrings (shown at left) 25–30 seconds each side; hip/glute, 25–30 seconds each side; quad/hip flexor, 25–30 seconds each side; IT band (sides of legs), 25–30 seconds each side; and calves, 25–30 seconds each side.
• If you have a partner who can assist you, a massage would include upper back, 25–30 seconds; upper trapezius, 25–30 seconds each side; and shoulder/upper arm, 25–30 seconds each side.

"iron out" knots that form in a muscle due to tension. This makes The Stick an effective relaxation tool for stress relief. Studies prove it: Self-massage using this device lowers cortisol levels, so indirectly, the technique can aid weight control and help you subtract body fat. Once you start incorporating self-massage into this program, you'll be amazed by the results.

Measuring Your Hormones
Stress Hormones and the Adrenal Stress Index

Chronic stress takes its toll on your adrenal glands, which produce the body's two stress hormones, cortisol and DHEA. If your stress is chronic, cortisol is released in larger-than-normal amounts. At the same time, the production of DHEA, which counterbalances the effects of cortisol, falls off. When these hormones become imbalanced, every part of your body can be adversely affected. Your immune system is compromised, for example, and this leads to increased risk of infection and disease. Even your body's use of glucose, along with insulin function, is altered causing higher blood sugar levels. You're likely to retain sodium and water, a situation that produces a tendency toward high blood pressure. Blood fats increase and predispose you to heart disease. The function of your thyroid becomes impaired, resulting in decreased metabolism, lowered body temperature, and reduced energy. Your body begins to store fat, especially around your midsection.

You can take a simple test to find out how your body's stress response system is functioning. It is called the Adrenal Stress Index (ASI), and it involves timed collections of saliva. The ASI gives a full profile of your cortisol levels throughout the day. You simply collect samples of saliva at certain points during the day, then send those samples off to a laboratory to get your results.

You can obtain a home test kit with your doctor's order, and lab fees are arranged through your doctor. The ASI is an excellent tool for identifying low adrenal function and a possible underlying cause for symptoms such as low energy, lack of libido, low blood pressure, low blood sugar, food and salt cravings, poor sleep, dry skin, depression, poor immune function, anxiety, and premature aging. Depending on the test results, you'll want to initiate a more or less aggressive approach to stress management.

Thyroid Hormone and the Thyroid Function Test

Everything from how readily your body burns calories to your mood is regulated by your thyroid gland, a butterfly-shape gland at the base of your neck that produces hormones which affect metabolism. As long as this gland manufactures the proper amount of hormones, your body functions normally.

If you're gaining weight even though you've been working out and following a healthy diet, you should have your thyroid level tested. An underactive thyroid, medically known as "hypothyroidism," slows down your metabolism.

The opposite, and less common, condition is overactive thyroid, or "hyperthyroidism," which can cause excessive weight loss. Thyroid function tests can be performed if your physician suspects a problem. If one exists, you'll be treated with prescription medicines.

Even though treatment of thyroid disease requires more than changes to diet and exercise, there are some lifestyle implications. For example, people with hypothyroidism can avoid weight gain or lose weight by choosing low-fat dairy products and meats and foods prepared with little or no fat. Someone with hypothyroidism would be wise to eat plenty of protein foods, such as dairy foods, fish, poultry, and lean meat, in order to build muscle.

Also vital for maintaining good thyroid function is exercise. It increases blood circulation to the thyroid gland and it decreases stress, thereby alleviating many of the symptoms associated with poor thyroid function, such as low energy and muscle and joint stiffness.

Remember to speak with your doctor about any possible thyroid issues, and if you are diagnosed with poor thyroid function, follow your doctor's orders to the letter.

Metabolism and Sleep

Fact: People who are sleep-deprived are more likely to be overweight than their well-rested counterparts. In one study, researchers at Columbia University and St. Luke's-Roosevelt Hospital in New York City analyzed data about the sleeping habits and weights of 18,000 adults between the ages of 32 and 59. What they found was intriguing: The people who got less than four hours of sleep each night were 73 percent more likely to be obese than were those who slept between seven and nine hours a night—the recommended amount for good health. There's more: Those who slept only five hours a night were 50 percent more likely to be overweight than those who slept seven to nine hours, and those who slept six hours were 23 percent more likely to be overweight.

Another study followed nearly 500 Swedish men for 13 years and found that less sleep was linked to a higher Body Mass Index (BMI), which typically correlates with excessive body fat.

Interesting don't you think? You're probably wondering exactly what the link is between weight and sleep. At this point scientists sum up their theories in one word:

hormones. When you're sleep-deprived your fat tissue decreases its production of leptin, a hormone thought to suppress appetite. Leptin production peaks at night when you're asleep. If you're not getting enough shut-eye, leptin production falls off. The less leptin that is circulating in your body, the greater your appetite, so you're prone to overeating and you're more likely to overindulge in tempting foods, whether it's junk food or easy-to-grab convenience foods.

In a study conducted at Stanford University, investigators studied 1,024 people who had participated in a research project called the Wisconsin Sleep Cohort Study. They found that people who habitually slept less than eight hours had higher BMIs than people who slept at least eight hours a night. Further, they discovered that shorter sleep times were associated with increased circulating ghrelin and decreased leptins, a hormonal pattern linked to obesity. Ghrelin is a hormone that stimulates appetite, fat production, and body growth.

Sleep deprivation also causes a drop in another hormone—human growth hormone—which is required for muscle development and fat burning. When growth hormone is in short supply, you can almost guarantee a metabolic snafu in which less fat is burned.

There is more to the hormone story: When you consistently get a good night's sleep, you allow other important hormones like melatonin and testosterone to be produced naturally and in greater amounts. When your body is sleep deprived, these hormones cannot be produced in the proper amounts. Lack of sleep also triggers your body to release higher levels of cortisol, a hormone tied to weight gain.

Losing sleep clearly changes your metabolism for the worse and sets the stage for weight gain. A study conducted at The University of Chicago discovered that a sleep debt of three to four hours over a few days was all it took to provoke metabolic changes that mimicked prediabetes. In the study researchers monitored 11 healthy young adults for 16 consecutive nights and found that when their sleep was restricted to four hours for six consecutive nights, their ability to stabilize blood glucose levels fell dramatically.

Sleep deprivation jeopardizes weight management and metabolism in another way. When you're feeling spent and fatigued all the time, you're less likely to work out regularly. This sets up the proverbial vicious cycle: poor sleep, poor motivation to exercise, slower metabolism due to lack of exercise … and so it goes.

There is a more simplistic explanation for the link between sleep and weight: The more time you're awake, the more time you have to eat. This may involve munching late at night when your metabolism slows a bit. What you eat at night is less likely to be burned off and more likely to be stored as body fat.

Whatever the explanation, it's clear that you need adequate sleep to maximize the metabolic process that burns fat and develops muscle. To look and feel your best, and keep your metabolism healthy, you require about seven to nine hours of quality sleep every night. So how do you make that happen?

Keep in mind that everyone has a sleepless night every once in a while. That's normal, and there are life situations that will temporarily disrupt our sleep patterns. After our daughter was born, my wife's and my sleep patterns were completely out of whack, since we had to get up at all hours of the night to tend to our newborn. I'm sure you can relate if you have children!

But if sleeplessness becomes more than occasional, this spells trouble and threatens not only your metabolism but your entire well-being, since poor sleep quality also harms your immunity and prevents your brain from rejuvenating properly. You may have fallen into the habit of sleep deprivation. Fortunately though, habits are learned behaviors—which means they can be unlearned.

Here are my guidelines for getting more shut-eye to maximize your metabolism:

- **Include natural, complex carbohydrates in your diet.** Follow the recommendations in my Nutritional Life Plan in Chapters 8 and 9. Carbohydrates boost serotonin, a brain chemical that relaxes your body and promotes better-quality sleep.
- **Maintain a healthy weight.** Use the *Make Over Your Metabolism* program to achieve this goal. If you're overweight, you are prone to sleep apnea, a potentially life-threatening condition characterized by loud snoring and brief interruptions in breathing during sleep, often hundreds of times a night. Extra pounds stress your respiratory system. Sleep apnea is also associated with atrial fibrillation, an abnormal heartbeat that increases the risk of stroke and heart attack. See your physician if you even suspect you may have sleep apnea.
- **Prior to going to bed, eat only *very* lightly.** Heavy meals or snacks eaten just before bedtime can interrupt your slumber. If you feel you need a snack close to bedtime, a very *small* piece of turkey is a good choice. Turkey contains tryptophan, a naturally occurring amino acid that enhances sleep and relaxation. You have experienced the effects of tryptophan if you've ever felt sleepy after having turkey for Thanksgiving dinner.
- **Get a minimum of three hours of exercise in each week.** However, be

sure to perform those workouts well before bedtime. Exercising too close to bedtime will lead to wakefulness because adrenaline and other hormones are elevated after exercise.

- **Watch your intake of coffee and alcohol.** Both interfere with sleep, so try to eliminate them or cut back.
- **Make sure your bedroom is restful.** A cool temperature, good ventilation, comfortable mattress or pillow, dark window shades, a room free of clutter—these all contribute to a sleep-inducing environment. On top of that, turn your mattress every three to four months to ensure maximum comfort for your entire body and a restful night's sleep.
- **Maintain a regular sleep schedule.** Go to bed and wake up at the same time every day. Your body will respond well to this kind of routine.
- **Try natural sleep-promoting tactics.** Take a warm bath before bedtime, use "white noise" (running a fan or sound spa), drink some chamomile tea, or put lavender aromatherapy oil on your pillow to induce relaxation.
- **Monitor your medications.** Certain types such as calcium channel blockers, steroids, decongestants, and caffeine-containing pain relievers can keep you from getting your zzz's. Consult with your physician and your pharmacist about your individual situation.

Everything Counts

Exercise and proper diet are not the only methods known to boost metabolism. Stress management and sleep quality are absolutely necessary to program your metabolism for fat loss so you can get slimmer and stronger and feel sexier. Give these weight-control methods a try—and watch yourself get fit and healthy for the rest of your life.

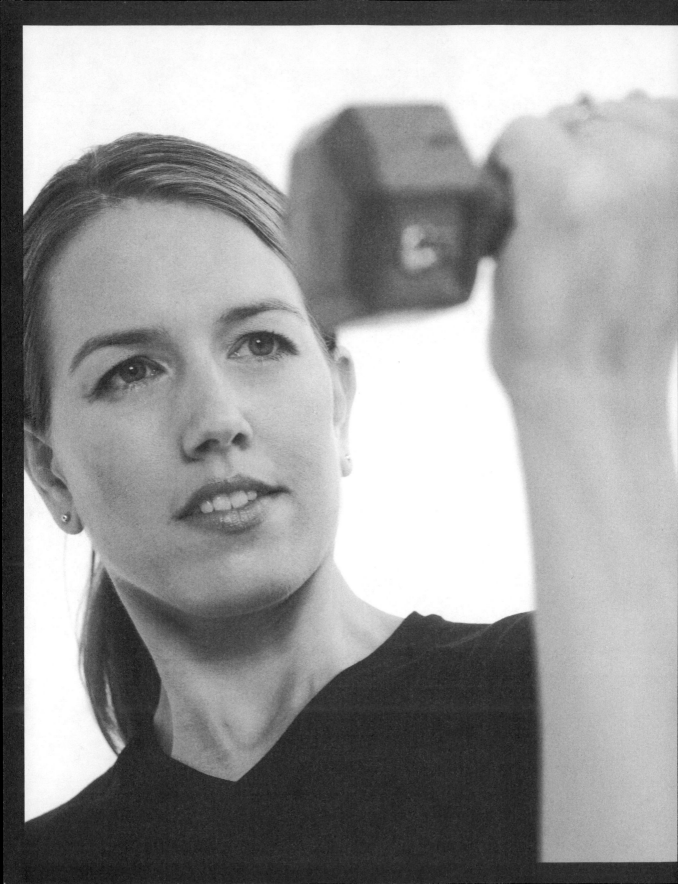

Chapter Three

FOUR MONTHS OF STRICT BED REST IN THE HOSPITAL BECAUSE OF A DIFFICULT PREGNANCY AND HEAVY MEDICATION HAD LEFT CARA ESPOSITO SO PHYSICALLY DEBILITATED THAT SHE COULD NOT WALK EVEN HALF A CITY BLOCK. HER metabolism was shot. The 34-year-old attorney decided to start training with me. She was determined to lose the weight she had gained during her pregnancy and regain her strength and stamina. Within eight weeks of training just three hours a week and following my Nutritional Life Plan, Cara made remarkable progress, almost against the odds. As she tells it, "Nine months after working with Robert, I was able to hike 10 full miles uphill in the Grand Tetons of Wyoming with no problem."

Shortly afterward Cara became pregnant again. And again she was put on strict bed rest, this time for six months. "After I gave birth to my second child, I was very worried that I would never get back into shape, especially with two kids and working as an attorney part-time," Cara says. "Where would I get the time? Thankfully, Robert has an amazing gift for making exercise easy. He made it fit into my life, not the other way around, and that helped my motivation so much. I am now thinner than I have ever been

Metabolic Motivators

in my life, including when I was in high school, and I am the strongest I have ever been."

One important point I must add about Cara: Like many people, she doesn't love exercise, and she admits she will go to great lengths to avoid it. Can you relate? But here's what she told me: "You have made it easy to include in my life, and I have stuck with it, which is a testament in and of itself to your program."

Staying the course with anything for the long term isn't easy. Exercise is no exception! Statistics tell us that six out of 10 Americans will drop out of their exercise programs within the first four months. Their initial motivation to exercise typically falls prey to a number of common excuses: not enough time, not enough energy, not enough interest. Given her attitude toward exercise and the complications with her pregnancies, Cara was a classic potential exercise dropout. But she was able to overcome her pessimism about exercising and start again, mainly because we worked on her *motivation muscle* too.

In this chapter you and I will train your motivation muscle so that you'll be mentally powered up to succeed. For you to be permanently successful with this program, your body and mind need to be in sync. Any positive change must begin with the conscious decision and desire to alter your old way of doing things, as well as devoting the necessary time and effort to achieve your goals.

Put Time On Your Side

The number one reason people give for not exercising, or for why they quit exercising, is time. Busy lifestyles, raising children, career demands, and personal obligations all

> I've been working with Robert for several years now. I woke up one morning very early on in our training, looked in the mirror, and said to myself, 'Holy @#$%, is that me?!' I've been hooked on Robert's work ever since. I'm 64 years old and have 10.5% body fat.
>
> **Michael O'Connell**
> INVESTOR VENTURE CAPITALIST
> HANCOCK PARK, CALIFORNIA

contribute to this problem. But it doesn't have to be this way. My *Make Over Your Metabolism* program offers solutions that won't stress your already busy schedule.

One of my promises in this program is that you won't overexercise but can get in shape with a minimum of three hours a week, even if that means 10- or 15-minute bursts of physical activity throughout your day. Such spurts of exercise can be just as beneficial— if not more—than one 30-minute workout. That means if you can't do your workout all at once, you can break up your exercise throughout the day. What counts as exercise? Lots of things. Walk fast to the office or grocery store. Take the stairs instead of the elevator. Walk during your lunch hour.

I want you to begin by committing to those three hours a week; that way you won't start out too rapidly and get burned out as a result. With good time management, everyone can squeeze three hours out of his or her week. Make your workouts a nonnegotiable priority, scheduling them on your calendar as you would any other important appointment. With a slight attitude adjustment, you can start thinking of exercise as a welcome break from other demands rather than as a chore.

Identify Exercise Benefits That You Value

With each workout you do, each healthy meal you choose, and each positive lifestyle move you make, you will feel the benefits. As those workouts, meals, and choices continue—in other words, as you develop consistency of effort—you'll begin to look and feel spectacular. Achieving a better appearance and higher energy level builds self-confidence. With exercise, healthy nutrition, and positive living, you can largely control how you look and feel. You really can. Think about it: In a world where so many things are out of your hands, here is something within your grasp: your body and, to a large degree, your health.

I'd like you to look at the list on page 58 and think about all the benefits of exercise, nutrition, and healthy lifestyle choices and decide which ones are most meaningful to you. Choose from the list or come up with your own. Post those benefits on your refrigerator door, on the bathroom mirror, in your car, or at your desk. That way you'll creatively work an awareness of your desire to get healthy into your everyday life. In a very short time, your motivation muscle will begin to get dramatically stronger.

Tune Out the Voice of Resistance

You've heard that voice in your head: "It's too cold outside. I'm tired. I'm too busy. I don't feel like driving to the gym." If you listen to it, your commitment goes out the

Health Benefits I Value Most

Review the list below and check off the health benefits that are most important to you. If you have others, add those to the list as well. Then make a copy of this page and post it on your refrigerator for daily inspiration.

☐ Faster metabolism

☐ More attractive appearance

☐ Pride in appearance

☐ Better weight control and management

☐ Improved flexibility

☐ Better coordination and balance

☐ Stronger immune system

☐ Extension of active lifetime

☐ Reducing reliance on medications

☐ Stress relief

☐ Delayed aging

☐ Less body fat

☐ Cardiovascular health

☐ Higher energy levels

☐ Greater endurance

☐ Better muscular development

☐ Lower blood pressure and resting heart rate

☐ Lowered cholesterol and other blood fats

☐ Clarity of thinking

☐ Improved bone health

☐ Improved sexual intimacy

☐ Better quality of sleep

☐ Enhanced self-esteem

☐ Better body image

☐ Self-confidence

☐ Ability to wear smaller sizes

☐ Looking great in clothes

☐ Preventing or controlling diabetes

☐ Setting a positive example for my children

☐ Reducing joint pain

window. Successfully motivated people manage to conquer that voice and develop other thought patterns that remind them how much they enjoy the benefits of working out and how important it is to exercise.

To conquer that negative inner voice, I recommend writing down the counterproductive thoughts. Alongside each statement write alternative, more positive statements with which you can replace the negative. Here are some examples below.

Turn a negative ...	... into a positive
I don't feel like driving to the gym.	But I want that workout that is going to give me the benefits I want, so today I will work out at home.
I've tried to exercise, but I always fail.	I don't always fail. Every healthy choice I make is a major success.
I'm too uncoordinated to exercise.	I'm gaining strength because I'm exercising. And I choose exercises that match my skill level.
I'm too fat.	Every moment I exercise and eat right, every time I make a positive health choice, my metabolism is becoming more efficient at burning fat for fuel.
I'm not very athletic.	Regular exercise makes me feel like the athlete I am.

I think you get the picture. The key here is to never be at odds with yourself regarding your workouts, your diet, or your health decisions. Always frame your thoughts both positively and rationally, because exercise, nutrition, and health are elements of your life that are to be cherished and honored.

> **❝** I've worked with Robert on and off now for almost 8 years. He has helped me recover from challenging injuries and provided a supportive but "excuse proof" environment. Something I dearly need! He has been key to keeping me strong and fit, despite my extremely time consuming and stressful career. His ability to perpetually motivate me (and have fun at the same time) never ceases to amaze me. What a wonderful magician! My family, clients, and I are all very grateful to him. **❞**

Sherry Grant
ATTORNEY AT LAW

What you're doing, in essence, is reprogramming yourself—you're retraining your motivation muscle. Your mind will be resistant at first, but you can counter that resistance with thought patterns that remind you how much you're getting from a healthy lifestyle.

Stop Holding On to Excuses for Failure

Recognize the sabotaging habits that keep you from succeeding. We all have them, whether it's drinking three beers a night or automatically helping yourself to seconds or eating too late at night. Be willing to give these habits up, or at least modify them, or substitute healthier actions. For example, if you find yourself wanting to dip into that tub of ice cream, do something else instead, something that is incompatible with over-consumption, such as walking your dog, going to a movie, reading a book, or exercising. Try to identify those habits that might be standing in your way, then take course-corrective action to minimize or eliminate them from your life.

Be realistic, however. Now and then you may return to some bad habits. You may even gain a pound or two. When it happens, don't be too hard on yourself. Simply get back on your program as soon as you can—with the next meal or the next workout. The only serious mistake you can make is to give up on your effort to change. Turn lapses into renewed

Emergency Foods

Keep some of these healthy foods on hand when you're on the road or stuck at your desk; they make a smart snack or a light meal. If you plan your daily meals appropriately—and take advantage of plastic containers and ice packs or coolers—you will rarely have to make food choices that will not service the goals in your Nutritional Life Plan.

Almonds

Walnuts

Tablespoon of peanut or almond butter in a small plastic container or bag (include celery sticks with this)

Various fresh fruits including apples, oranges, pears, peaches, apricots, grapes, cherries, raspberries, blueberries, figs, tangerines, plums, and strawberries (refer to pages 210–211 on Nutritional Life Plan Sanctioned Foods)

Wasa crackers

High fiber or whole grain cereal in a plastic bag

Various veggie sticks such as carrots, celery, zucchini, and pea pods

Hummus or nonfat dips for vegetables (use vinegar and olive oil or nonfat sour cream with spices)

Piece of whole grain bread or gluten-free bread

Various legumes (carry in a plastic container)

Whole grain tortillas or pita bread (add a teaspoon of almond butter or peanut butter, if you like)

Ground flax meal in a plastic bag

Low-sodium lunch meats, turkey, tuna in a plastic bag (carry with an ice pack)

Leftover meat choice from the day before (carry in a plastic container with an ice pack)

Hard-boiled eggs (carry in a plastic container with an ice pack)

Nonfat or low-fat yogurt (carry with an ice pack)

opportunities for improvement. Think about why a lapse occurred, take corrective measures, and then move on. Maybe there was leftover pie in the fridge, and you indulged because you let yourself get too hungry. A client of mine recently blew her program when she had to pick up her daughter from college on a moment's notice and ate fast-food sandwiches and french fries while on the road. This woman went into frantic mode over this, so we analyzed the situation to figure out the genuine cause of this little lapse. The cause was not having her "emergency food" with her. (Emergency food is healthy food that you *always* have with you in case you get hungry so you don't overindulge in the wrong foods.) Have emergency food, like some almonds and a piece of fresh fruit, available to you wherever you go and this will never be an issue for you. The lesson in this: Figure out why you lapsed, then take corrective measures so that it is less likely to happen again. In doing so, you'll come back stronger than ever!

Do It for You, Not for Anyone Else

It's well-known that to achieve long-term success, motivation must come from within rather than from outside influences. As soon as you feel controlled by demands or expectations from others, you can lose the motivation to continue on your own. You must express a genuine, deep desire—not one imposed by others—to look and feel your best. Being at your best lets your family and friends receive the very best of you.

Think about what I'm saying here. You are never being selfish by taking the time to work out and care for yourself. Your children, your spouse, your significant other, your friends, your pets, and everyone in your life will benefit from your *being the best of you,* prolonging both your longevity and quality of life. This is really important. And again, it's not about what you *need*; it's what you *want*. I encourage you to look closely at what I say on page 75 regarding the defining moment in your life when you became inactive. Examine what happened and move forward. There are options in *Make Over Your Metabolism* for everyone. Because this is about *your* "personal best," your goals are guaranteed to be within your reach.

So please do not make changes or start this program to please anyone else. Your loved ones will benefit automatically. Make this about you. Tell yourself that you're doing this because your body and your soul want to.

Excuse-Proof Your Environment

I believe strongly in making your environment work for you so that your motivation muscle stays strong. This is pretty simple to accomplish. Some suggestions:

- **Lay out workout clothes and equipment before going to bed.** You'll be less likely to talk yourself out of exercising in the morning.
- **Rid your home of junk food.** Have on hand only healthy foods, such as those recommended on my Nutritional Life Plan.
- **Schedule your workouts as you would a business meeting.** This is an appointment with yourself that will bring you closer to attaining and surpassing your goals while having fun along the way.
- **Make the effort to set up your own home gym.** Use the information provided in Chapter 4 and in the appendix of this book. Or if you prefer to go to a gym, choose one near your home that is easily accessible so you'll be less likely to miss workouts.
- **Read additional articles and books on exercise, nutrition, and fitness.** Increasing your knowledge of fitness helps build and maintain your motivation muscle.
- **Do the *Make Over Your Metabolism* program with a partner.** Studies show that people are more successful in adhering to an exercise or diet plan when they do it with others. You're less likely to duck out of an exercise session if your partner is counting on you to be there. But if your partner doesn't show up or starts to waver on the commitment, *you* must stay on track without missing a beat.

Keep a Fitness Journal

Research shows that recording your meals, snacks, and exercise activities in a fitness journal, as well as charting your progress, is a proven way to stay focused and build your motivation muscle. It keeps you accountable. To help you I have included a sample journal page in the back of this book. Make copies of this page to create your own fitness journal. Follow these guidelines to use it to your best advantage.

- **Write down your exercises, how many sets and repetitions you did, plus what kind of resistance you used.** For the cardio portion of this program, record your speed, time, distance, peak heart rate, and recovery heart rate. The fitness journal in the back of this book includes all of these categories.
- **Review your previous entries to keep yourself psyched up.** Before each workout, look at what you accomplished during your last workout. Decide how much you intend to do this time and what you'd like to improve, and

try to beat the last workout's personal best. Acknowledge all progress and success in your journal. Seeing your progress in black and white, and charting it over time, is terrific motivation and can be personally inspiring. You'll be surprised and uplifted when you see that you're getting stronger, building more endurance, and, of course, dropping the body fat like crazy! You can look back and say, "Wow, I'm tackling my goals. I'm succeeding. I'm getting in shape!" And the proof is not only in the mirror or on the scales but in your fitness journal.

- **Chart other information.** I think it is a great idea to track other details of your lifestyle too, such as how much sleep you get at night, how you handle stress, how you avoid some temptation, what works and what doesn't, and what your energy levels are during and after workouts, as well as throughout the day. Did you feel like you really accomplished what you wanted to this week? How do you feel about your accomplishments? I want you to really expand on how you feel, physically and emotionally, by writing in this journal.

  This sort of information is useful if you ever find yourself at a standstill because you may be able to pinpoint what is holding you back. Once you identify what is stalling your progress, you're on your way to correcting it.

  Also make notes about how your metabolism is changing. Signs that it is higher include steady weight loss and fat loss, looser-fitting clothes, greater perspiration during your workout, and greater intensity and level of effort during exercise.

> Do this program and change your life! Robert Reames is the master of the well-rounded and efficient workout. You will feel better and get stronger right off the bat!
>
> ## Tom Freston
>
> PRESIDENT AND CEO
> VIACOM, INC.

Be Good to Yourself

As you work through and meet each physical challenge on this program, incorporate the Nutritional Life Plan, and implement all the metabolism-enhancing guidelines, give yourself a well-deserved reward, such as a massage, a new outfit, or a special gift. Rewards leave happy associations in the mind—and set you up for more victories ahead.

Never, ever beat yourself up because you didn't achieve the level that you did last week. As long as you follow the program from week to week, you are succeeding. If you pulled your exercise equipment out of the closet and got to work, you are succeeding. If you ate a healthy lunch today, you are succeeding. If you got your eight hours of sleep last night, you are winning. It is all a process, and a positive process at that. Just do and be the best that you can every day.

If you're heavy right now and you've been heavy for a long time, you've probably been putting yourself down for a long time. Change that view right now. You are doing something incredibly positive for yourself, so don't bring in any negative vibes. There is no losing here, except for losing inches and body fat. You will win on this program *by implementing* the program. So please start thinking of yourself as the winner that you are.

Finally, Stay Positive

Keep positive energy flowing through your mind and body with daily affirmations. This will keep your momentum building. For example, tell yourself: "I have a strong, healthy body" or "I feel more energetic" or "I can see and feel my shape changing for the better." Visualize how you want to look after you've lost weight and firmed up on this plan. There is an old saying: "Whether you think you can or you can't, either way you are right." Make exercise, nutrition, and proper lifestyle choices positive experiences, and they will continue to reward you for the rest of your life.

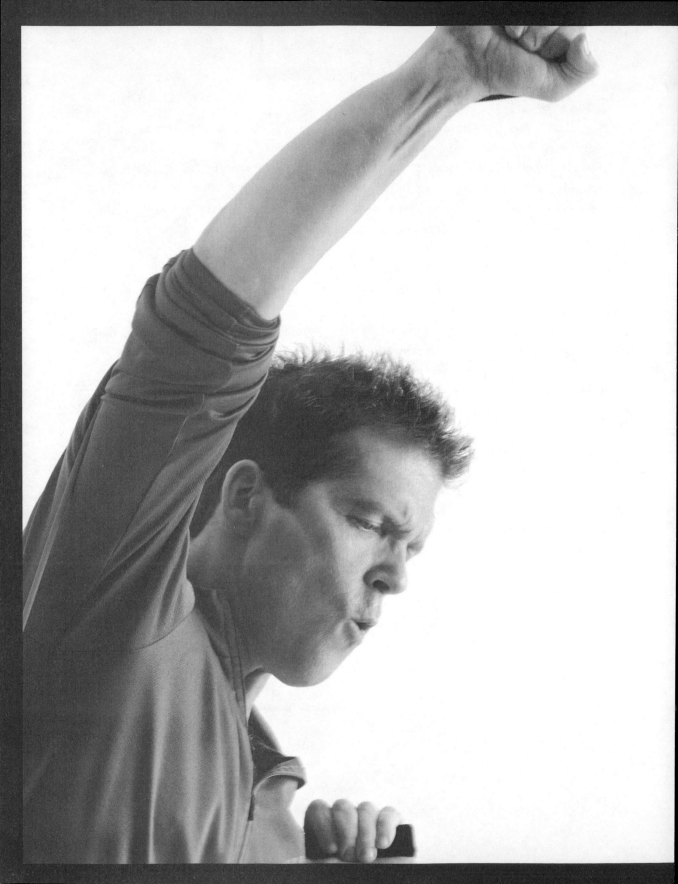

Chapter Four

I T'S TIME FOR TRUE CONFESSIONS. WHEN IT COMES TO EXERCISE, DO YOU VIEW IT AS ALL WORK AND NO FUN? LOSE INTEREST EASILY? GIVE UP BEFORE YOU GET THE RESULTS YOU WANT? IF YOU ANSWERED "YES" TO ANY OF THESE QUESTIONS, YOU are like a lot of people. As you prepare to start the *Make Over Your Metabolism* program, I want you to know your attitude plays a huge role in your fitness plan. "Attitude" is the way you approach or view a situation. Most people approach exercise as work, when they would be better off approaching it as play—play that has a purpose. If you learn to love the three hours a week you spend exercising, achieving your goals will be easier and more enjoyable.

You are about to find out how to make exercise fun, how to bring back the kid in you who used to like to play, romp, and compete. One of the keys to enjoying your workouts is to compete against yourself and pursue *your* personal best. Get in the habit of asking yourself every day: "How great can I look?" "How strong can I get?" "How fast and how far can I walk, jog, bike, swim, or run?" Athletes ask themselves these questions all the time as they push past their previous limits and strive constantly to attain their personal best. There *is* an athlete in every one of us.

Getting in Gear

Our first step in bringing out that athlete will be to find out where you are now in your fitness journey. How is your general health? How much do you weigh? What are your goals? How many inches would you like to lose? What dress or pants size would you like to wear? How fit are you right now? Before you begin taking your metabolism, your body, and your fitness to a higher level, you need a personal baseline assessment against which you'll measure your continuous progress.

Preparticipation Checklist

It is always wise to check with your physician before beginning any type of exercise program or nutrition plan. Your doctor can zero in on any conditions that might limit your participation. He or she will be very pleased that you took this step and will offer you even more encouragement for putting the information in this book to work in your life. In fact, I think it is a good idea to inform all of your health care practitioners about your quest to attain and maintain your optimum metabolism.

As a personal trainer, I always give potential clients a health and medical questionnaire and require that their physicians approve their participation in my program. You'll find a condensed version of that questionnaire on the next page. It is not meant to diagnose any medical condition nor to take the place of an examination by your physician. However, it can alert you to potential problems or help verify that you're fit enough to participate.

Baseline Weight, Body Fat, and Circumferences

As you begin the *Make Over Your Metabolism* program, have a specific, realistic weight goal in mind. In other words, you must shoot for a weight at which you will look and feel your best. Keep in mind that there is no such thing as the "perfect" weight because people come in a variety of body shapes, heights, and bone structures. There are, however, ideal weight ranges, and these can be determined through a very simple calculation. For example, to determine the midpoint of a woman's ideal body weight range, allow 100 pounds for the first 5 feet of your height, and add 5 pounds for each extra inch.

If you're within 10 percent (lower or higher) of that midpoint, you're within your ideal weight range. The lower end of the range is for small-boned individuals; the upper end is for larger-boned people. To make this easier for you, see page 70 for two charts showing ideal weight ranges for women and men (with the midpoints in bold).

You should weigh yourself once a week to check your progress toward your weight goal. You will want to monitor your progress in another way too: by using a simple tape measure and taking body circumference measurements each week of your hips, thighs, and

Preparticipation Questions   **Answers**

1. Has your doctor ever informed you that you have heart trouble?   Yes ☐   No ☐

2. Have you ever been diagnosed with diabetes?   Yes ☐   No ☐

3. Has your doctor ever said your blood pressure was too high or too low?   Yes ☐   No ☐

4. Has your doctor ever told you that you have arthritis or another joint problem that could be aggravated by exercise?   Yes ☐   No ☐

5. Do you now or have you ever smoked?   Yes ☐   No ☐

6. Are you taking any prescription medications?   Yes ☐   No ☐

7. Have you had any major illnesses or surgeries within the past two years?   Yes ☐   No ☐

8. Could you be described as "sedentary" and not accustomed to exercising?   Yes ☐   No ☐

9. Are you older than 35?   Yes ☐   No ☐

10. Is there a good medical reason not mentioned here why you should not engage in an exercise program?   Yes ☐   No ☐

If you answered "yes" to any question, please consult with your doctor before starting any exercise program.

abdomen. Set realistic goals for these measurements as well and prepare to watch the inches melt away as you continue on this plan.

While measuring, stand with your feet together, breathe normally, and keep your abdomen relaxed. Do not take measurements over your clothes. The tape measure should be snug on your skin but not constrictive. Take the following measurements using a cloth tape measure:

1. Your waist at your naval
2. Your waist approximately 1 inch above your naval
3. Each thigh at its widest point
4. Your hips at their widest point

Record these measurements weekly. This first assessment provides the benchmark against which you'll measure your progress toward a firmer, shapelier you.

An optimum way to monitor your progress is by measuring your body fat percentage using a home scale called a "bioelectrical impedance scale." Your body fat percentage is considered to be a very accurate look at how much actual fat you're losing. The scale analyzes body fat as a standard feature, along with weight. It works by measuring a signal it sends through your body. A faster signal means you have more muscle on your body. That's because water conducts the signal, and muscle is about 70 percent water; fat contains little water, so it impedes the signal. A body fat range of 18–25 percent is generally considered healthy for physically active women; for men, a healthy range is from 10–18 percent.

Use the handy scorecard on page 71 for recording your measurements:

Ideal Weight Ranges for Women

Height	Ranges	Height	Ranges	Height	Ranges
4' 11"	85-**95**-105	5' 4"	108-**120**-132	5' 9"	131-**145**-160
5' 0"	90-**100**-110	5' 5"	113-**125**-138	5' 10"	135-**150**-165
5' 1"	95-**105**-116	5' 6"	117-**130**-143	5' 11"	140-**155**-171
5' 2"	99-**110**-121	5' 7"	122-**135**-149	6' 0"	144-**160**-176
5' 3"	104-**115**-127	5' 8"	126-**140**-154	6' 1"	149-**165**-182

Ideal Weight Ranges for Men

Height	Ranges	Height	Ranges	Height	Ranges
4' 11"	90-**100**-110	5' 6"	128-**142**-156	6' 1"	166-**184**-202
5' 0"	95-**106**-117	5' 7"	133-**148**-163	6' 2"	171-**190**-209
5' 1"	101-**112**-123	5' 8"	139-**154**-169	6' 3"	176-**196**-216
5' 2"	106-**118**-130	5' 9"	144-**160**-176	6' 4"	182-**202**-222
5' 3"	112-**124**-136	5' 10"	149-**166**-183	6' 5"	187-**208**-229
5' 4"	117-**130**-143	5' 11"	155-**172**-189	6' 6"	193-**214**-235
5' 5"	122-**136**-150	6' 0"	160-**178**-196		

My Measurements

	Weight	Waist (at navel)	Waist (above navel)	Right Thigh	Left Thigh	Hips	Body Fat %
Starting Measurements							
Measurements at 1 Week							
Measurements at 2 Weeks							
Measurements at 3 Weeks							
Measurements at 4 Weeks							
Measurements at 5 Weeks							
Measurements at 6 Weeks							
Measurements at 7 Weeks							
Measurements at 8 Weeks							
Measurements at 9 Weeks							

My Goal Weight: _____ Goal Pant Size: _____ Women: Goal Dress Size: _____

Personal Fitness Assessment

Next I would like you to take some easy tests to determine your baseline fitness levels in the areas of endurance, speed, strength, and balance. This is valuable information to have at the onset of the program. Record it on the scorecard on page 73. You can use the results to periodically evaluate your progress in each area. I suggest that you retake each test every four weeks. If you've followed the program to the letter, you should see a noticeable improvement in your scores and feel more energized and confident about your abilities. Imagine how motivating and affirming it will be to see yourself improve as you continue to raise the bar and constantly increase your fitness level. Plus, as you become more fit, the pounds and inches will just keep coming off, bringing you closer and closer to your realistic goals and beyond!

You can perform these assessments virtually anywhere, including your own backyard, at any time with minimal equipment. You will need these:

- A stopwatch (a watch with a second hand will do)
- A standard chair
- A solid wall
- A calculator and tape measure (if you are manually measuring a 1-mile course)

Keep in mind that the assessments you are about to take are measurements of your *current* fitness level. You are not out to set any world records. Your objective is simply to do your best. Use good sense and be mindful not to exceed your limitations on the given day. If you feel pain at any point during the assessment, stop immediately. Pain is your body's method of communication. Exercise should not be hazardous to your health; safety is the number one concern with any fitness activity.

Warm-Up

Before taking this fitness assessment, warm up your muscles by exercising on a cardio machine or walking for five to 10 minutes.

1-Minute Wall Push-Up Test

This exercise tests your upper-body strength and muscular endurance (the ability of your muscles to resist fatigue). You'll need a sturdy wall and a stopwatch (or a watch with a second hand). Do as many push-ups as you can in one minute. Get your entire body involved, not just your upper body. Use the scorecard on the next page to record the number of push-ups you were able to complete in one minute.

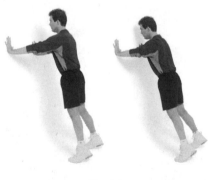

To perform this test correctly, follow these instructions:

- Place the palms of your hands against the wall, directly in front of your shoulders. Fully extend your arms.

Test	Date:_____	Date:_____	Date:_____	Date:_____
1-Minute Wall Push-Up Test Score				
1-Minute Chair Squat Press Test Score				
1-Mile Test Score	Time_____	Time_____	Time_____	Time_____
	Distance_____	Distance_____	Distance_____	Distance_____
Single-Leg Balance Score	Right___ Left___	Right___ Left___	Right___ Left___	Right___ Left___

- Draw your belly button in toward your spine while maintaining normal breathing. Do not let your back arch excessively.
- To execute the motion, bend your elbows to no more than a 90-degree angle. Return to the starting position. As you perform the wall push-up, keep your body in one straight line—don't let it waver.
- Record the number of push-ups you complete in one minute.

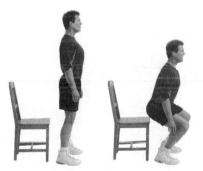

1-Minute Chair Squat Press Test

This exercise tests your lower body strength and your muscular endurance. You'll need a standard chair and your stopwatch. Use the scorecard above to record the total number of chair squats you are able to complete in one minute.

To perform this Chair Squat Press Test correctly, follow these instructions:

- Stand in front of the chair. Place your feet a little farther than shoulder width apart. Stand nice and tall with your arms positioned comfortably at the sides of your body. This is the starting position.
- To execute this motion, bend your knees to no more than a 90-degree angle, as if you are going to "sit" in the chair. Do not exceed the range of motion that is comfortable for you.
- Return to starting position and repeat.
- Record the number of chair squat presses you complete in one minute.

73

1-Mile Test

This exercise measures your endurance and stamina. You can perform the test on a premeasured track at a school, health club, or YMCA. Or you can use any safe open space, such as a large parking lot, a park, a schoolyard, a city block, or a tennis court (23 times around a regulation tennis court equals one mile). If necessary, measure the distance of the space you plan to use with the odometer in your car or bike. A tape measure and a calculator may also be useful for measuring distances. Your goal is to set up a 1-mile course. Remember: 5,280 feet equals 1 mile; so does 1,760 yards. Be sure to have your stopwatch with you.

In this test, you'll travel 1 mile as quickly as possible by walking, jogging, or running. Remember that this is a baseline fitness assessment. Do not attempt to exceed your limitations. This testing is part of an overall assessment that provides you with the data to track your improvements and progression over time. I recommend that you walk your initial 1-mile test. If you need to rest along the way or if you need to stop all together, that's okay too. Do the very best that you can *today*.

To perform this test, follow these tips:

- Determine your 1-mile course.
- Use a stopwatch or a watch with a second hand.
- On your mark, get set, go! Cover the 1-mile distance as quickly as you can. Feel free to walk, jog, or run. But, again, do not exceed your limitation or expect to perform to standards you cannot yet achieve on the very first day. Rest along the way if you need to and stop at any point if you feel you cannot make the entire distance.
- Record your time and the distance traveled.

Single-Leg Balance

This test evaluates balance—how well you can maintain stability during daily activities and exercise. Having good balance helps prevent falls, especially as we get older.

To perform this test, follow these smart tips:

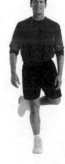

- Make sure the area is free of hazards that you could potentially fall against or trip over.
- Stand nice and tall on one leg. Stay in this position as long as possible, up to 3 minutes. Repeat on the other leg.
- Record the balance time for each leg.

Think back ...

When I was a kid, we didn't have computers, video games, and all the other electronic entertainment we have now. We played tag, ran races, swung on swing sets, and played basketball (a lot of basketball in Indiana!). Kids are hardwired to enjoy active experiences like these! My mother had to rope me to get me home for dinner. My 6-year-old daughter is no different. She and her friends are like Energizer Bunnies. Even kids who are not as athletic keep going and going just for the sake of having fun. Playful activity is something all kids love; it's natural and it's good for them.

Remember your own childhood, when you were engaged in active play and having the time of your life? When did that stop? Was it in fifth grade when you didn't get picked for the kickball team at recess? When a kid laughed at you because you didn't have the greatest athletic skill? When someone called you "fatso" one day? When you got too involved in computer games and got lazy? When you had an injury in high school? When you put on that "freshman 15" at college? When a car accident prevented you from being active? Were you unable to shed the weight gain from pregnancy and just gave up? Or did you just decide at some point that play wasn't a priority, that your "adult" responsibilities did not leave time for fun and exercise?

My real question: Why does physical activity ever have to stop? There is a defining moment or time in every inactive person's life when he or she disallowed the kid inside from having fun and stopped being physically active. I believe it is critical to define that moment in your life, acknowledge it, learn from it, and move on to find activities that you authentically love to do. Give yourself permission to have fun physically!

Physical activity increases not only your longevity but also your quality of life. This is no big secret. When you're active you feel better about yourself because you have energy. Your body takes on a healthier shape, which renews your self-confidence. You're in control of your life. The bottom line is that healthy choices make you a winner in every aspect of your life. You owe it to yourself and your loved ones to make the most of your life!

Exercise Toys

Let me help you take the first step toward enjoying exercise by introducing you to some inexpensive, easy-to-store "exercise toys" that you will be using on this program. Working out with these pieces of equipment—a stability ball, dumbbells, elastic tubing, and a medicine ball—gets you back to the fun, playful aspect of exercise. On top of that, these toys can form the basis of your very own home fitness facility.

They are truly toys—toys with a purpose. If you walk into a gym or workout room, the spaces look like recreation rooms, filled with colorful balls, jump ropes, and other toylike devices. I have found that when my clients start thinking of these tools as toys with a purpose, they begin to enjoy their workouts more and become very engaged in the time they spend exercising. And this equipment is downright fun to use!

If you are intimidated right now by the thought of going to a gym, exercise toys are the perfect solution. You can start exercising in the privacy of your own home and not have to deal with a lot of complicated-looking equipment, at least not at first. You can indeed make over your body without ever leaving the comfort of your house. Anything you can accomplish at a gym can easily be re-created at your home or office without sacrificing the quality of your workouts. The type of workout these exercise toys provide is just as challenging as any gym routine, as long as you use the tools effectively.

Our bodies perform, function, and benefit the same wherever and whatever the workout venue. We push, pull, press, and rotate, regardless of where we are. Exercise toys let us incorporate and enhance these same movements. Further, they train our bodies by employing multijoint movements. In other words, you're getting more muscles involved than you would in just single isolated moves. Multijoint movements activate, stimulate, and develop more lean muscle tissue for a faster metabolism, plus they improve your body's ability to operate as a unit. The more muscle you build and develop, the higher your metabolism will be. More fat is thus burned, and it's burned 24-7! With the minimal amount of time you invest in your workouts, you're getting greater results and more for your investment.

You do not need to purchase all the toys right away. You can use equipment that you already have and purchase as much as your budget allows. (For help on setting up a home gym that fits your space and budget, see the Appendix, starting on page 246.) Several of the workouts in the *Make Over Your Metabolism* program make use of exercise toys such as a stability ball, dumbbells, exercise tubing, and medicine balls. Before you choose the workout that best fits your needs, here is an overview of how the toys work.

Elastic Tubing

Elastic tubing is made of flexible, stretchable rubber and has handles on the ends for comfort and easy use. You can use these bands to work any muscle group, including triceps, biceps, chest, back, shoulders, thighs, glutes, hamstrings, and abdominals. Upon setup of a given exercise, tubing follows your body movement. This provides you with "made-to-order" exercises that adapt to the way your body is structured. In contrast, when you use weight machines, your body has to adapt to the motion of the machine.

Exercise tubing comes in several resistance levels, which are determined by the elasticity and denoted by color. The exercises in *Make Over Your Metabolism* are freestanding, so all you'll need is your tubing and you—no door attachments or the like. You can use tubing at home, while traveling, or at the gym.

Stability Ball

The stability ball, a.k.a. the body ball, physio ball, exercise ball, or Swiss ball is a staple in the exercise world. Ball training originated as a mode of rehabilitation in Europe and became popular in the United States in the 1960s. It's here to stay. No home gym or public fitness facility should be without at least one unit of this most versatile and effective piece of exercise equipment.

Like most exercise toys, a stability ball is relatively inexpensive and offers an astronomical return on your investment. There are stability ball exercises for weight loss, strength conditioning, balance, toning, core stabilization, muscle building, muscular endurance, sports-specific work, and overall body conditioning.

Performing exercises on the ball places your body in an environment that is unstable. This calls many of your muscles into play to provide your body with necessary stability, coordination, and balance. As a result, you develop muscles more effectively, enhance balance, and make your body less prone to injury.

Stability ball training also allows you to maximize your exercise experience, giving you a strong musculoskeletal foundation and enhancing all activities of daily living as well. Most work done on the ball requires a great deal of recruitment from your core muscles, and this contributes immensely to better posture and body alignment, as well as a faster metabolism.

Stability balls come in different sizes and inflations. Be sure to select one that's right for your height so you'll derive the most effectiveness from the exercises. The chart below gives important guidelines.

- For exercisers shorter than 5' 0", choose a 45 cm ball.
- For exercisers between 5' 0" to 5' 8", choose a 55 cm ball.
- For exercisers between 5' 9" to 6' 3", choose a 65 cm ball.
- For exercisers taller than 6' 3", choose a 75 cm ball.

Pumping more air into the ball increases the efficiency of use for a given exercise. A less inflated ball has a "mushy" feel and can make the exercises more difficult to execute properly. Proper body positioning is also an important component. The exercises you learn will teach you how to position your body correctly for best results.

Dumbbell Free Weights

Dumbbells are small, compact, and short. They typically come in pairs and range in weight from 1 pound to 100 pounds. Free weights have been a mainstay in exercise programs forever. Free weights are effective; they enable you to do the work of body sculpting and body development, plain and simple. Free weights build and develop the active, fat-burning muscle that you want to maximize your *Make Over Your Metabolism* program. Some dumbbells are adjustable, meaning you can change the poundage on the bar and secure the weight with a special device called a collar. However, to save time and make your workouts as efficient as possible, I recommend fixed-weight dumbbells, which can be purchased in sets or one at a time. Fixed-weight dumbbells don't require that you spend precious time changing the weights and resistance levels. Filled water bottles and cans of food can be used as free weights as well. Thus you can succeed on any budget.

Medicine Ball

Your grandfather might have worked out with a medicine ball, an exercise tool that was patented in the 1890s. It did not become popular, though, until after Herbert Hoover became president of the United States in 1929. Although an active outdoorsman, Hoover ballooned to 200 pounds after taking office. His physician invented a new game with the medicine ball to reduce Hoover's presidential girth. The medicine ball remained a favorite training tool in the first half of the 20th century, until athletes found it more fun to play basketball and volleyball.

Today the medicine ball has rebounded as an exercise toy (with or without handles), available in weights ranging from 2 to 20 pounds. Medicine balls free your body to twist, turn, and toss. They are a great way to target the core and integrate your total body into each exercise.

They're effective for sports-specific training too. They supply resistance as you go through the same motions used in golf, baseball, basketball, and volleyball, to name a few. The medicine balls also work effectively for what I like to call "life-specific" motions that emulate the functional movements we make in everyday life. You can work alone or toss a ball back and forth with a partner.

Indoor Cardio Unit

On my program you'll be performing a special type of cardio exercise called "Metabolic Burst Training," explained in more detail in Chapter 5. This work is a key element in boosting your metabolism 24-7 so that you can successfully manage your weight, lose inches, continuously transform your body, attain your realistic fitness goals, and maintain the optimal overall health and wellness that you desire and deserve.

Metabolic Burst Training does not need to involve the purchase of any special equipment. It can be done at the YMCA, the mall, and in and around your home, depending on the activity. You can incorporate it into walking, jogging, running, swimming, biking, or any movement that you choose for physical activity anywhere, anytime. However, you have the option of using the cardio equipment at the gym or purchasing your own cardio machine for home use. Here is a brief overview of three of the most popular cardio exercise machines used in fitness centers and home facilities worldwide.

Treadmills

Walking, jogging, and running have been staples in exercise programs since the beginning of time, so it's no surprise that treadmills provide an excellent weight-bearing workout. Walking and running are natural motions, and treadmills provide a smooth, very predictable terrain—no rocks, chuckholes, or uneven surfaces. Most treadmills on the market today provide flexible decks as well. This means you'll get a safe and comfortable workout.

Elliptical Trainers

Elliptical trainers combine the motions of a treadmill, stepper, ski machine, and bike in one nonimpact, weight-bearing motion. Some elliptical machines provide both forward and backward motion for variety. Total body elliptical trainers provide arm motion as well. If you work on a unit that does not have the arm motion equipment and you make natural arm movements on your own, you'll gain balance and core training benefits. Be ready to hold on to the handrails (try not to lean on them) should you need to catch your balance or rest.

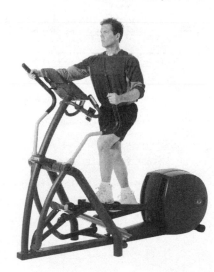

Stationary Bikes

Upright bikes *(pictured near right)* take up very little space and have provided both fun and fitness for many people over the years. They provide a non-weight-bearing form of cardio exercise, but that does not mean the workout lacks intensity. Ask anyone who has trained for a bike race! Recumbent bikes *(pictured far right)* offer the comfort of added back support. Comfort is not synonymous with laziness in this case. After all, you

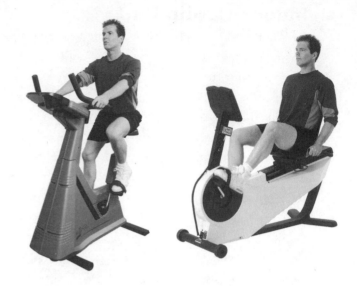

control your intensity level. Because the legs are more level with the torso on a recumbent bike, the blood return back to the heart through your veins is very efficient. The lower body workout from either type of stationary bike is excellent.

Pedometers

This is a must-have! If you're looking for extra motivation to move, I recommend a pedometer, which increases your awareness of your activity level and helps you see the progress you're making on this program. This small, inexpensive device clips to your waistband and counts your steps. Think of it as a little personal trainer.

A study in the *International Journal of Obesity* found that people who take at least 9,000 steps a day are more likely to be classified as normal weight, while people who take less than 5,000 steps are more likely to be classified as obese. In another study 400 women ages 19–71 were encouraged to walk 10,000 steps a day for eight weeks and to wear a pedometer while doing so. By the end of the experiment, nearly half of the women reported losing weight. Those who set daily step count goals also said they improved muscle tone, increased their energy, fit into their clothes better, and decrease stress.

Start wearing a pedometer as you go about your day. Once you know how many steps you usually take, you're ready to set goals. (Most people take anywhere from 2,000 to 5,000 steps per day.) Aim to add 2,000 steps every day until you hit 10,000 (which is equivalent to approximately 5 miles and burns 400–500 or more calories a day).

If you take 10,000 steps, you'll walk about 5 miles. Tall people cover more distance in fewer steps than shorter people. That's OK. No matter whether you're short, tall, or average height, your goal to maximize weight loss should be at least 10,000 steps per day. This amount is a very realistically achievable goal to attain on a daily basis.

As you increase your daily activity, you increase the amount of calories and fat you are burning, plain and simple. It's fun to track your steps with a pedometer, and it is a clear indication of the amount of movement you get throughout your day. If you are on the move and busy burning calories, then you won't have time to overeat or lead a sedentary lifestyle. So keep on walking!

One note: The surgeon general recommends getting a minimum of 30 minutes of physical activity per day to help lower blood pressure, decrease body fat, and increase cardiovascular fitness levels. You'll achieve this amount by following the *Make Over Your Metabolism* program, so the steps recorded on your pedometer are a bonus built in to your day. Record these steps in your journal. It all adds up and it all counts!

Heart Rate Monitors

I strongly recommend using a heart rate monitor when performing Metabolic Burst Training and resistance training. These monitors indicate your heartbeats per minute (bpm) and are one of the best ways to monitor your individual exercise intensity, as well as to track your progress. As you progress in your cardio workouts, you will see that you can do more work with less effort. (For more information, see Heart Rate Monitoring, page 154.)

Take the Next Step

If you've done the work of this chapter, you're ready to begin the *Make Over Your Metabolism* exercise program. Remember, focus on achieving your personal best each time you work out: the specific resistance you want to work with, the intensity you want to put into Burst Training, and most of all, having fun while you're working out.

Imagine it is one month from today, and you've stuck to the plan. Ask yourself: How will my life be different? How will it feel to look at myself in the mirror? How will it feel to fit into smaller clothes? What kind of compliments will you be receiving? Calling to mind feelings of success in the future creates passion today. And passion translates into the motivation you want and need to live healthfully every single day. You deserve that kind of lifestyle. It belongs to you. Now it's time to go after it.

It only gets better from here.

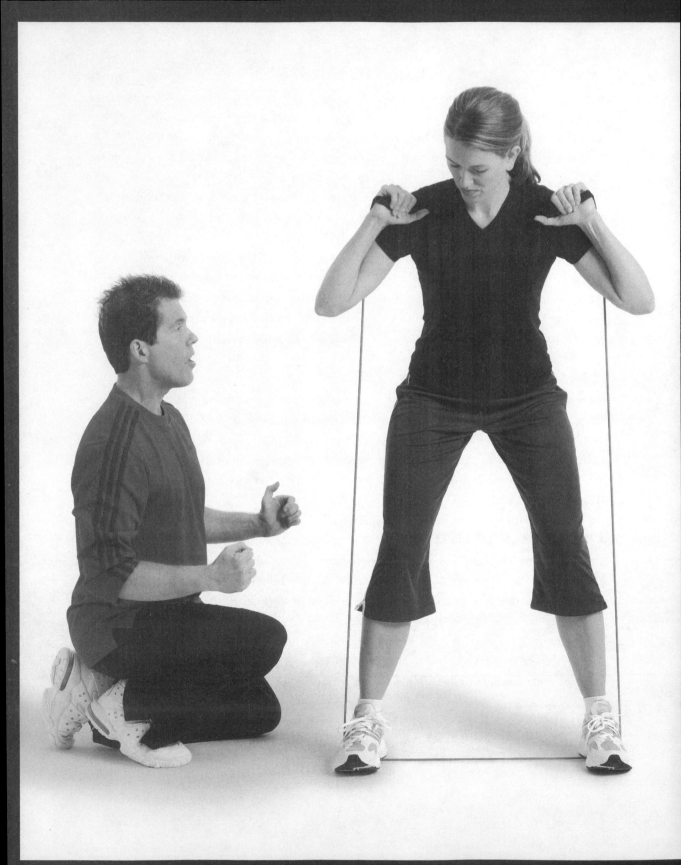

Chapter Five

I CAN'T TELL YOU HOW MANY PEOPLE ARE SKEPTICAL AT FIRST ABOUT THE IDEA OF GETTING IN SHAPE IN JUST THREE HOURS A WEEK. THEY SAY, "OH, COME ON, CAN YOU REALLY DO THAT?"

You absolutely can follow an effective workout plan in just three hours a week! In fact three hours a week not only makes sense if you have a busy schedule, but the latest studies show that it is plenty of time to get in shape. That's because of the metabolic after-effect, or "afterburn," of working out. Just 30 minutes of exercise a day maximizes your metabolism for the remaining 23.5 hours. You burn more calories and fat while you sleep, drive your car, get your kids ready for school, work at your computer, and even eat, all *as a result of this training.* This is in addition to the fat and calorie burning that occurs *during* your workout as well. You do, in essence, become "a fat burning machine"!

As long as you stay consistent and continue to raise the bar on both your resistance and Metabolic Burst Training workouts, you will discover that working our three hours a week is plenty of quality time to reap a host of fitness benefits that include the following:

Make Over Your Metabolism Basics

- A change in body shape from fat to firmness
- Enhancements in strength
- Improvements in stability, flexibility, and posture
- Upgrades in your energy system and work capacity
- A recharged and revved-up metabolism

You can get those results by doing 30 minutes of resistance training, which includes a two-minute maximum intensity bout of cardio three times a week, and 30 minutes of Metabolic Burst Training three times a week. Each workout winds up with a few minutes of calming stretches to restore hormonal and mental balance. This all adds up to only three hours a week. On this plan you must commit to those three hours each week and fit them into your schedule. Team this physical training with my Nutritional Life Plan and my easy-to-implement lifestyle tips, and the result will be lean, attractive muscle, a fast-charged metabolism, and success in achieving your permanent fat-loss goals.

When you give those three hours your all, you can get your body in the best possible shape. You can beat the unfairness of your currently slower metabolism. And you can get off the seesaw of weight gain and weight loss. You'll be able to get your body in gear to speed up your metabolism and start losing inches and pounds—and do it so that fat burning practically goes on automatic pilot.

The *Make Over Your Metabolism* plan is divided into two four-week programs. In the initial four weeks—the beginner program—the focus is on building a fitness foundation that burns lots of calories, raises your metabolism, and builds body-firming muscle that will allow you to maintain optimal calorie burning all day long.

After the initial four weeks, you will intensify your total body workouts in the advanced program by adding two new exercises designed to build strength and balance. You also have the option of implementing any of the specialty programs you'll find in Chapter 7. These exercise routines are designed to "spot-condition" trouble areas such as your thighs, hips, abs, lower back, and upper body.

On top of that, you will begin to amp up your Metabolic Burst Training after the first four weeks. If you've been walking I'll encourage you to take it up a notch in the second four weeks to jogging or running. If you've been doing a non-weight-bearing activity, such as biking, you may be ready to incorporate a weight-bearing activity into some of your workouts during the second four weeks. You may be swimming, and now you're ready to try biking, a treadmill, or an elliptical trainer. Regardless of what activity you are doing, this will be the time to raise your individual exercise intensity to the next level. You may be ready to attempt a group class such as kickboxing or aerobic dance at a gym, recreation center, or YMCA. Explore your opportunities. By changing your routine or "revving it up" to the next level, you'll begin to realize your fitness potential and experience how much better your body can perform.

Resistance Training

I know that you want what we all want from exercise: more body-firming muscle and less unsightly fat. When you do resistance training, you build and develop lean, precious, active, valuable fat-burning muscle, which is a highly metabolically active tissue. Muscle is the most effective calorie-burning tissue in your body. Recall what I said earlier in this book: Muscle is like having a brigade of fat-burning fireplaces throughout your body. As you continue your resistance training over time, more fireplaces ignite and the existing fireplaces become more intense. Not only do you burn more calories when you work out, but more important, these fireplaces are working to burn fat 24-7! By continuing to build and develop muscle, you kick your metabolism into high gear.

Let me again clarify that this phenomenon takes place all throughout the day, even though you don't actually feel the burn. It's going on beneath the surface, at the level of your cells and tissues. For every pound of muscle you develop, your body burns an additional 40–50 calories per day—and that burn happens even during times of rest and total relaxation. It's like a great investment that keeps the cash coming in around the clock. Muscle dictates metabolism. Muscle runs the show.

In Chapter 6 I will take you through the four-week workout plans, exercise by exercise, just as if I were standing right next to you as your personal trainer. I'll guide you so that you will know exactly what to do at each step along the way. But first let's talk about the terminology and principles behind the workouts so you'll understand why the *Make Over Your Metabolism* program is so effective at changing your body into a better fat-burning machine.

The Push-Pull System

The motions of pushing, pulling, pressing, and rotating form the foundation of any resistance training program, whether you are a beginner or an elite athlete. Most of the exercises in my plan involve a push-pull system. Basically this means that you work a pushing muscle group, followed by a pulling muscle group. There are two major advantages to exercising in this manner.

First, a push-pull system trains your body functionally in a way that's consistent with how you naturally move and live. Think about the simple action of pulling open your car door. You don't just use your fingers and arms to perform the task; you use your back, traps, rhomboids, rear delts, obliques, and a whole bunch of other muscles all at once. In other words, your body works as a unit to execute such "life-specific" motions. A push-pull system helps you develop overall strength that can greatly enhance your daily life activities.

Second, with a push-pull system, you train muscle groups equally to keep your body in balance, which helps prevent injury. If you over- or underwork certain muscle groups, you can create an imbalance around your joints. The underworked muscles and connective tissue become lax and lengthen, while the overworked muscles shorten and become tight. Such imbalances can lead to tendonitis, stooped shoulders, and lower back problems, just to name a few. A push-pull system helps to prevent muscular imbalances.

Multijoint Movements

Most of the exercises in the *Make Over Your Metabolism* program involve multijoint movements, meaning they don't work just one body part in isolation but several together. And they hit your body's largest muscle groups. Multijoint exercises increase the fat-burning potential of your muscles because the movements require more energy and access and stimulate more muscle per exercise.

Squats, seated rows, and push-ups are examples of multijoint exercises. They comprehensively access several large muscle groups at one time. The seated row, for example, calls into play the muscles of your back, rear shoulders, core, and biceps.

By contrast, movements only at one joint (often called "isolation exercises"), such as arm curls and leg extensions, use up valuable time and work less muscle. Compare the isolation exercise motions with the multijoint action of a bridge or squat press. You'll see and feel the greater payoff of using more muscle in each exercise. I'm not saying that you should never do single-joint isolation exercises; some areas of the body warrant special attention, and we'll go over that in Chapter 7. But if you want to get in shape in the shortest time possible, plus increase your metabolism, focus your energy on working as much muscle as possible in every exercise. Multijoint exercises stimulate the maximum amount of muscle tissue in the least amount of time per workout. Result: You work more muscle, and your metabolism works faster and better. In other words: more payoff for the time and effort you put in. The metabolic benefits for fat loss are indisputable.

Multijoint exercises also build stability, the basis for most of the movements you do every day, from walking down the street to toting luggage to the airport. If you have a strong foundation and center, you'll not only look better but also be more efficient at your movements, which will improve your exercise performance, decrease your potential for injury, and help you enjoy a better quality of life.

The 7 Acute Resistance Training Variables

You can modify or manipulate the following variables in your resistance training to make the most efficient metabolic and body-shaping gains.

1. Number of sets. A set is a certain number of repetitions performed in sequence without stopping for rest. A repetition (or "rep") is one complete movement of any exercise within the set from start to finish. You will add sets to your workout during the course of the first and second four-week plans. If you have never lifted weights before, begin with one or two sets of every exercise listed for the first week and progress to two, three, or even four sets in the second, third, and fourth weeks.

2. Number of reps. Generally you'll perform 10–15 repetitions per set. Chapter 7 is very specific about how many repetitions to perform of each exercise, eliminating any doubt or confusion.

3. Resistance. Resistance is the amount of weight or challenge from your own body weight or from tubing. Resistance stresses your muscles sufficiently to promote development. You'll hear me say this a lot: *Resistance levels must be comfortable, yet challenging.*

Select a weight or resistance that will challenge you. If you fatigue, give out, or "really feel it" between repetitions 8 and 12 while maintaining good form on the exercise, you've picked a good resistance level. If after three or four reps you're screaming for help, you've used too much resistance. Any pain that you feel in a joint while you're performing a rep is a signal to stop and lighten your level of resistance. Remember, pain is your body's method of communicating that something is wrong. If you can zip through 12 or more reps before feeling any twinges of muscle fatigue, the resistance is too light.

The key is to effectively challenge your muscles to the best of your own ability, performing each repetition with optimum form and safety. You may be able to manage 10 or 12 repetitions with a 10-pound dumbbell, while someone else performs the same number of reps with a 5-pound dumbbell.

You'll continually add resistance as you get stronger. This stimulates your muscles in fresh ways and prevents plateaus. As you progress beyond both plans, you will continue to build and master more exercises to keep your workouts fresh and challenging.

4. Intensity. Intensity refers to how hard you work out. For a muscle to continue developing, you must work out harder and harder, which may mean increasing the resistance, the number of repetitions, or the number of sets. Intensity also involves variations in the speed at which you perform each repetition—doing them super slowly or speeding them up. That doesn't mean you increase the total time you spend working out. Whether you do eight, 12, or 15 reps in a set, you should reach what's called "failure"—the point where you can't do another rep without breaking form. That's maximum intensity.

5. Form. Form is the way you position your body, your path of motion, and the way you perform the motion while moving through an exercise from beginning to end. To get the most out of every repetition, it is crucial to use proper form. Focus on using controlled movements, particularly on the descending or return phase of each exercise. I highly recommend that you practice each exercise without any resistance at first in order to perfect your form. You're sacrificing proper form if you find yourself "throwing" a weight, relying on momentum to perform the work for you, or losing control and rushing through a set. These actions can compromise your results and lead to injury.

6. Rest periods. Minimizing the rest period between sets maximizes fat loss. Incorporate a 30- to 45-second maximum rest period between sets. In other words keep on the move; don't waste time or rest too much. Make the most of your exercise time and think positive flow and momentum. Transition rhythmically from one set to the next, from one exercise to the next, training at your highest level of intensity on a given day. Following your resistance training, you flow right into two minutes of maximum intensity cardio work prior to your cooldown of calming stretches at the end.

Shorter rest periods are associated with metabolic advantages. For one thing, a workout paced with shorter rest periods maximizes your hormonal response. In a recent exercise study, one group of volunteers took one-minute rest periods between sets, while another group took 30-second rest periods. The hormonal response was measured in both groups, and the results were intriguing. Levels of growth hormone and two other fat-burning hormones—epinephrine and norepinephrine—were higher in the exercisers who took the 30-second rest periods. What's more, the short-rest exercisers got stronger and increased their muscular endurance. It all goes to show that just one small adjustment in how you work out—such as taking shorter rest periods between sets—pays big dividends in terms of your metabolism.

Maximizing your hormonal response helps promote lean muscle, body fat reduction, strong connective tissue, and even youthful skin and appearance. That's one of the reasons I view resistance training as a "fountain of youth." The ability to manipulate your overall hormonal responses like this is another key reason why the *Make Over Your Metabolism* program works so effectively.

7. Frequency. I know I keep harping on this, but you don't have to spend hours and hours at the gym or in a workout room. The resistance training part of this plan (see the workouts in Chapter 6) is to be done a minimum of three days per week on nonconsecutive days, such as Monday, Wednesday, and Friday, or Tuesday, Thursday, and Saturday. This gives your muscles time to rest, remodel, and recover so they're refreshed and ready to perform the next workout.

For perspective, this off-the-clock recovery period is when the muscle development takes place, so rest is really important to your metabolism. It sounds like a contradiction in terms, but when you let your body recover, it responds by developing lean muscle. Thus my philosophy is to work out very hard and rest well.

A Word About Your Warm-Up

The warm-up at the beginning of your workout basically prepares your body for physical activity. It promotes active blood flow to the working muscles, increases heart and respiratory rate, raises overall body tissue temperature, and prepares your nervous system to call your muscles into action. Proper warm-up gets you *ready* for action and will help ensure a quality workout. Your warm-up should last approximately five to eight minutes, and should involve the following:

- 4–5 minutes on cardio equipment of your choice, marching or jogging in place, and/or walking around the premises such as your house, yard, office building, or neighborhood
- 10 seconds of arm circles to the front and 10 seconds of arm circles to the back
- 12 high knee lifts (alternate 6 per side)

Activating Your "Supercenter"

In most of the exercises, I will ask you to activate your "supercenter," also known as your "core." Your supercenter—the area around your trunk and pelvis—is where your center of gravity is located, and it's there that all movement in your body originates. When you have good strength and stability in your supercenter, the muscles in your pelvis, lower back, hips, and abdomen work in harmony. Like a strong pillar holding up a building, they support your spine for just about any activity. When the muscles of your supercenter are hard at work, they keep you upright, stabilize your body as your weight shifts, absorb impact from ground forces, and help other muscle groups move more effectively.

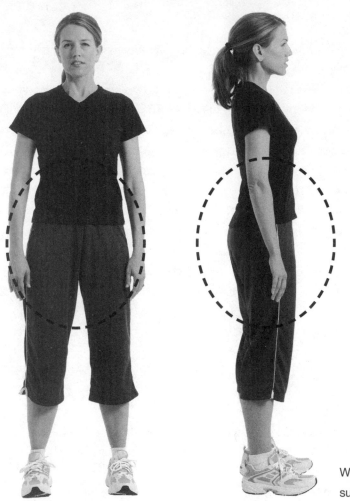

We all have a
supercenter!

This enhances the foundation of the exercises, improves your posture, and builds core strength and stabilization for better function and independence. With a strong super-center you can function better in all aspects of your daily life, whether it involves carrying your toddler or a bag of groceries.

If your supercenter has become weak over time, you are susceptible to poor posture, injury, and lower back problems. Developing a strong supercenter helps correct or even prevent these issues.

To activate your supercenter during resistance exercises, draw your belly button in toward your spine and stand, walk, or sit nice and tall while maintaining normal breathing.

Metabolic Burst Training

In addition to your resistance training routine, you'll do cardio work. No, I'm not talking about 60 to 90 minutes of floor-pounding aerobics or training for a marathon. I'm talking about Metabolic Burst Training, a special form of cardio that will complement your resistance training and maximize your body's all-important fat-burning response.

A "burst" is a brief bout of higher-intensity activity, such as a sprint, alternated with a period of lighter exercise. Keep in mind that when I use the word "sprint," it's a relative term. You'll do your sprint at your own best level of intensity, and this level will constantly improve as you continue on this program. For the first eight weeks of the *Make Over Your Metabolism* program, you'll perform bursts in one-minute intervals.

Your burst may be walking faster around your neighborhood or at the mall. Or it may be increasing the incline on your treadmill. Maybe you walk the hallways at work or at home, and your burst may be to incorporate intervals of running up and down the stairs.

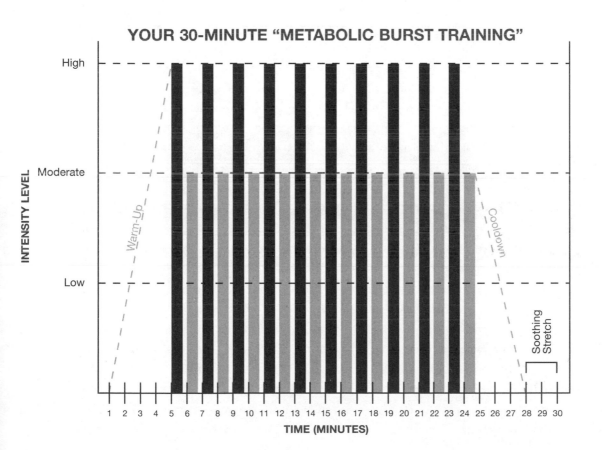

YOUR 30-MINUTE "METABOLIC BURST TRAINING"

You might run all out for one minute, then walk or jog for one minute. Other examples would be a one-minute sprint in the pool followed by one minute of a swim at a more leisurely pace. Your sprint may be a faster pace on the bike or the use of a higher resistance level. Or your sprint may *actually be an all-out sprint.*

My point is that your "sprint" is the maximization of *your* level of work for your chosen activity. You can use this short-burst interval method on any type of equipment at any location—from the schoolyard or the office to an airport.

The newest information we have shows that Metabolic Burst Training is superior to conventional aerobic exercise for weight loss, fat loss, and overall improvements in body composition. For one thing, it releases hormones that stimulate lean muscle development and promote a higher calorie burn. Metabolic Burst Training burns fat without wasting any of your precious muscle for energy, as prolonged aerobic exercise is prone to do. In fact, bursts are advantageous to your muscles. They exert force just like resistance training does and therefore train your muscles to grow stronger.

Excessive cardio work (I'm talking hours upon hours) will not help you achieve your weight loss goals more quickly unless you're willing to depend on this type of approach forever. Nor will it necessarily give your body the definitive curves and shape you want. To understand what I mean, visualize a sprinter or tennis player, both of whom do high-intensity short-burst training in their sports, standing next to a long-distance runner, who trains daily with hours and hours of exhaustive running. Athletes who perform high-intensity, short-burst training tend to have well-shaped, nicely muscled physiques, while some long-distance athletes, though thin, can often look stringy.

Don't get me wrong—there is nothing wrong with long-distance running as a fitness pursuit or sport. It is superb conditioning. However, a large volume of research shows that shorter interval "sprint"-type training is overall more beneficial for heart and lung health than moderate-intensity cardio exercise done over long distances or for long durations. However, intermittent bursts of cardio, like my Metabolic Burst Training, produces additional benefits. Two of these are better body composition (a favorable proportion of metabolism-boosting muscle to fat) and increased metabolic afterburn. And whereas conventional aerobics like long-distance running improves aerobic endurance (the ability to keep moving aerobically without fatiguing), Metabolic Burst Training improves both aerobic endurance *and* anaerobic endurance (the ability of your muscles to sustain intense, short-duration activity such as weight lifting or sprinting). In everyday life, what this means is that as a result of this training you will increase your ability to sprint through an airport to catch a plane if you're running late or make a beeline to a store in the mall to get in on the 50-per-cent-off sale before the store closes!

My point is that you don't have to put in the hours that a long-distance runner puts in to get in shape. There are more productive uses of your time that yield faster and better results by keeping your metabolism optimally elevated 24-7, and those are the exercise, nutrition, and lifestyle methods I'm focusing on in this program.

Excessive cardio also will raise stress hormones and eventually break down your muscle for energy. I believe that there is no extra benefit to extending the duration or time of your cardio work. (For additional cardio workout options, see "Beyond the First Eight Weeks: More Metabolic Burst Training Options," page 203.)

Realize that the intensity of your work is your primary concern in the *Make Over Your Metabolism* program. You will be stronger on some days than on others. This is all part of the process that absolutely everyone, even the most elite athlete, experience. But the important message here is to continue reaching *your* highest level of intensity during a given day's workout. You are taking positive steps every day—and this makes every day a success!

You want to maintain and continually develop muscle to optimally enable your body's ability to perpetually burn fat. When you add Metabolic Burst Training to your exercise mix, you make huge strides in losing fat and reshaping your body. Remember, you're guiding your body and gearing your metabolism to run optimally off the clock and not to be dependent on hours of exhausting, muscle-wasting, and time-*inefficient* daily marathons of cardio.

It's Time to Start!

So take a deep breath and set aside every notion you've ever had about exercising. You are about to get your body in shape, your health in line, and your metabolism running so efficiently that the pounds and inches will seem to melt away. You'll start feeling positive about yourself because you are in control of your health destiny, maybe for the first time ever. All you have to do is follow me for the next eight weeks and watch the contours of your body change for the better.

OK, what are you waiting for? Now's your chance to get leaner, firmer, and healthier and to feel sexier and more attractive!

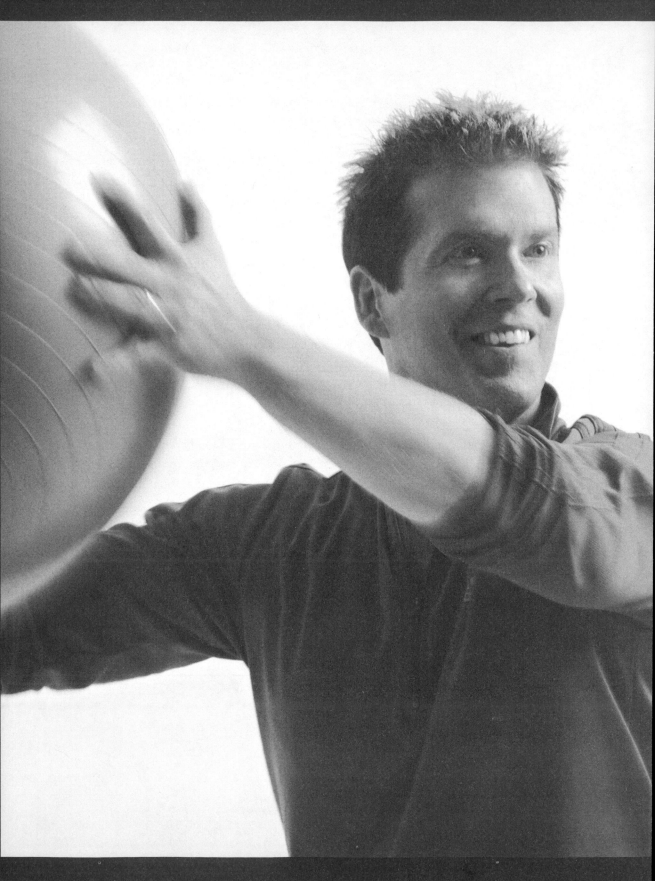

Chapter Six

B EFORE I STARTED WORKING WITH MONIKA BARKLEY, WHO WAS ONE OF THE PARTICIPANTS ON DR. PHIL'S *Ultimate Weight Loss Challenge*, SHE HAD NEVER DONE RESISTANCE TRAINING AS PART OF HER REGULAR EXERCISE, EVEN when she was active. For 20 years, she battled yo-yo dieting and overate when she felt depressed and overwhelmed. Food was a constant in her life, a "drug" of choice. As a result her weight spiraled up to 197. She was 42 and unhappy.

Through the *Ultimate Weight Loss Challenge*, Monika achieved her goal weight of 142, losing 55 pounds. Her body composition changed at an incredible pace once she began following my *Make Over Your Metabolism* workouts—which are all focused on resistance training—and doing Metabolic Burst Training. "Robert ramped up my fitness program to a new level that I never thought my body could endure," Monika said. "He helped me to realize a potential that I never could have believed for myself."

Today, at 44, Monika sports a body with 18 percent body fat, wears a size 4, and loves it. She's thrilled with her new self-image and is equally grateful for how energetic she feels and how much the changes have improved her relationship with her husband, Sam.

Make Over Your Metabolism Workouts

Monika's story exemplifies what can be achieved when you shift your metabolism into high gear and let it go to work for you. She took responsibility for making that happen with the right combination of exercise, healthy eating, and revamping of her lifestyle.

The same dramatic changes can happen to you, and they can be permanent, as long as you, too, make my *Make Over Your Metabolism* Workouts, Metabolic Burst Training, Nutritional Life Plan, and simple lifestyle tips a part of your life. The programs I'm about to outline are the first steps in elevating your metabolism to optimum levels 24 hours a day. The more consistent you are, following these programs very closely, the more positive changes you will notice. Your clothes will fit better, the number on the scale will move down, the inches will come off, and your energy levels will skyrocket.

Before we get to the actual workouts, here is how the exercise program works.

You have four beginner workouts to choose from for the first 4 weeks of the program and then four advanced workouts to try in weeks 5–8:
- Tubing and Body-Weight Workout: Beginner, page 100
- Tubing and Body-Weight Workout: Advanced, page 112
- Chair and Dumbbell Workout: Beginner, page 118
- Chair and Dumbbell Workout: Advanced, page 124
- Stability Ball and Dumbbell Workout: Beginner, page 130
- Stability Ball and Dumbbell Workout: Advanced, page 138
- Gym Workout: Beginner, page 140
- Gym Workout: Advanced, page 148

With the first six options, you can work out in your home; with the last two options, you can work out at a gym. Make your choices based on the exercise equipment and venues (home, office, fitness center) available to you. All of the workouts follow the same general pattern. Each lasts approximately 30 minutes and should be performed three times a week on nonconsecutive (alternate) days. You'll begin to see and feel results very soon, and you'll be amazed at what such short workouts can accomplish.

In the following pages I've provided photos and instructions for the exercises in each workout option. Some exercises are included in *every* option. Follow the workout you have chosen one exercise at a time, in the exact order I have listed. *Complete all sets of one exercise before moving to the next exercise.* I recommend that you have this book with you as you train. I want you to feel as if I were right there with you as your own personal trainer, guiding you through each exercise and congratulating you on your great work.

A Note on Breathing

Maintain normal breathing throughout each exercise. Exhale on the initial motion (pushing, pulling, squatting, pressing, or rotating) and inhale on the return phase. Never hold your breath during any part of an exercise.

Squat Concerns

The squat, or what I am calling Squat Press in the *Make Over Your Metabolism* program, is the most comprehensive lower body exercise the human body can perform. It accesses and stimulates the largest muscle groups of your entire body all at one time—which of course results in more manufacture of fat-burning machinery. Talk about value for time! Plus the Squat Press is one of the most functional, or what I call "life-specific," exercises you can perform. It is a must-do exercise if you're on a quest for permanent fat loss.

You may be leery of this exercise—and quite validly so—if you have back, knee, hip, or ankle issues. Please speak to your physician if you have concerns.

This movement is a part of daily life: when you get in or out of a chair or a car, squat down to get a pan out of the bottom cabinet, pick up your toddler, put wood in your fireplace, climb stairs, kneel down to tie your shoes, go to the floor to fix something, or pick up something to move it or put it in a higher place.

In this book you are learning the correct and safe way to perform this exercise; this will help you incorporate the motion properly in your daily life, as well as help you better manage your weight. When performing a squat, your main concerns should be the *range of motion*, the *path* of motion or total form, and the *resistance levels* being used. The motion in and of itself is natural. On page 121, I demonstrate a Basic Squat Press with a limited range of motion that may be comfortable yet challenging enough for you at the beginning. If you've never done this exercise before, I strongly recommend that you place a chair or bench behind you; it'll give you a sense of security and guarantee that you're performing the exercise with correct form because sitting is a familiar motion.

If you absolutely do not want to perform this exercise for now, then add two more sets of the Chair Bridge (page 105). Incorporate the Squat Press when the time is right and you feel comfortable doing it.

Major Muscle Groups of the Body

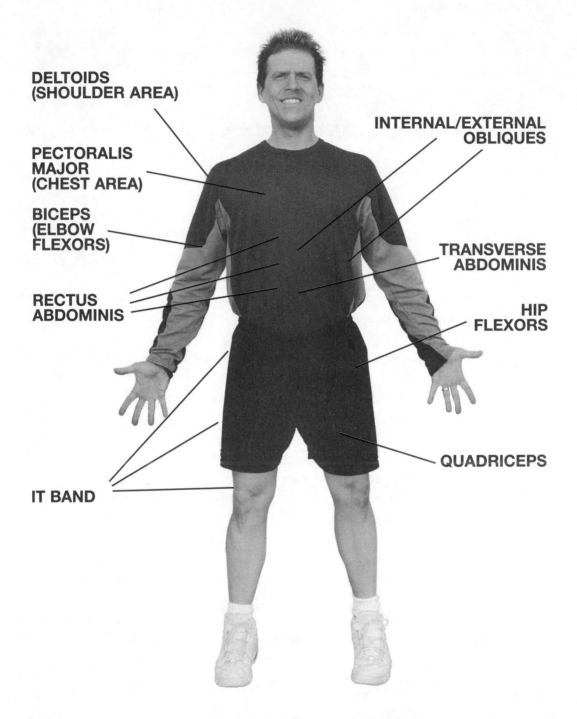

DELTOIDS
(SHOULDER AREA)

PECTORALIS
MAJOR
(CHEST AREA)

BICEPS
(ELBOW
FLEXORS)

RECTUS
ABDOMINIS

IT BAND

INTERNAL/EXTERNAL
OBLIQUES

TRANSVERSE
ABDOMINIS

HIP
FLEXORS

QUADRICEPS

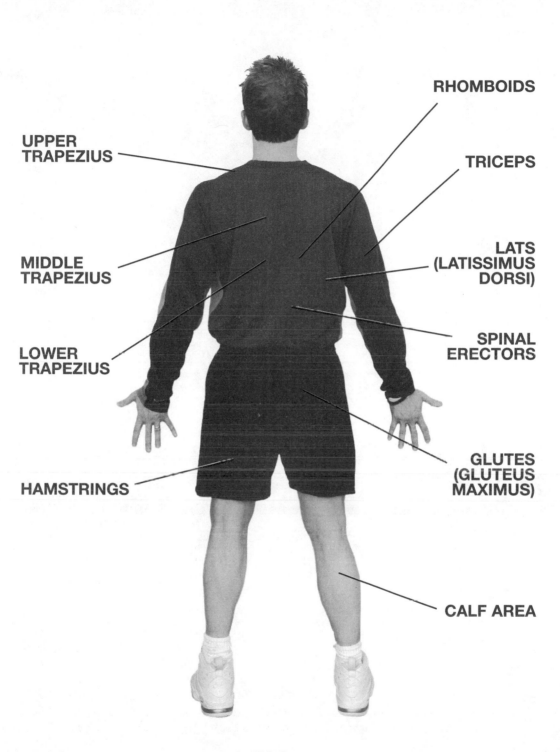

RHOMBOIDS

TRICEPS

UPPER TRAPEZIUS

LATS (LATISSIMUS DORSI)

MIDDLE TRAPEZIUS

SPINAL ERECTORS

LOWER TRAPEZIUS

GLUTES (GLUTEUS MAXIMUS)

HAMSTRINGS

CALF AREA

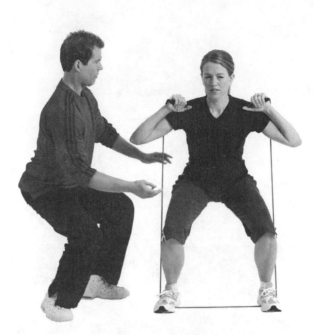

BEGINNER
Tubing and Body-Weight Workout

This is the first option you can choose for your
Make Over Your Metabolism workout. This is a simple workout
you can do most anywhere, whether you're at home or on the
road. The tubing is inexpensive and portable. Before starting
this program, read the safety guidelines on the next page.
Then get started by following the workout on the following
pages. After 4 weeks, you can move up to the "advanced"
portion of this workout, which immediately follows these pages.

WARM-UP
•4–5 minutes on cardio equipment of choice, marching in place, or walking around •10 seconds of arm
circles to the front; 10 seconds of arm circles to the back •12 high knee lifts (alternate 6 per side)

ROBERT'S RULES FOR TUBING SAFETY

•Do not store your exercise tubing in extremely hot or cold environments or in sunlight. Don't let your tubing get wet.

•Before each use, check your tubing for cracks or holes or any loosening of handles. Run your fingers and hands across all aspects of the tubing to check for deformities. If your tubing is damaged, replace it immediately.

•Keep your tubing away from sharp objects.

•Tubing is to be used only for specific exercises. Please keep it out of the reach of small children.

•Keep the handles away from your face and never perform any tubing exercise directly toward your face.

•Maintain your balance during tubing exercises. Keep your feet properly spaced with your knees bent to ensure maximum stability.

•Only one person should use a piece of tubing at a time.

•Do not combine or tie two pieces of tubing together.

•Do not overstretch your tubing; this could damage it.

•Clear your workout area of any potential obstacles. You want to have plenty of floor and air space to complete your exercises.

•Wear proper footwear to exercise. Avoid high heels and shoes with cleats.

1. STANDING TUBING CHEST PUSH

Target: Chest, shoulders, triceps, balance, and core

Positioning: Stand nice and tall in a slight lunge position, keeping both feet firmly planted and your knees slightly bent. Activate your supercenter.

Secure the tubing by placing it underneath the arch of your back foot. Grasp the tubing handles and hold them slightly to the side in front of your shoulders with your elbows bent, as shown. Align the tubing just to the outside of your body and not between your legs.

Motion: Extend your arms overhead at approximately a 45-degree angle toward the ceiling, as shown. (Notice that the path of motion is not straight ahead, but not directly overhead either.) Extend your elbows to neutral at the top of the motion. Do not lock your elbows. Return to the starting position and continue the exercise for the recommended number of repetitions.

Tip: If this exercise presents pain or discomfort in your back, neck, or shoulder area, you may substitute the Wall Push-Up on page 72 or the Knee Push-Up on page 119.

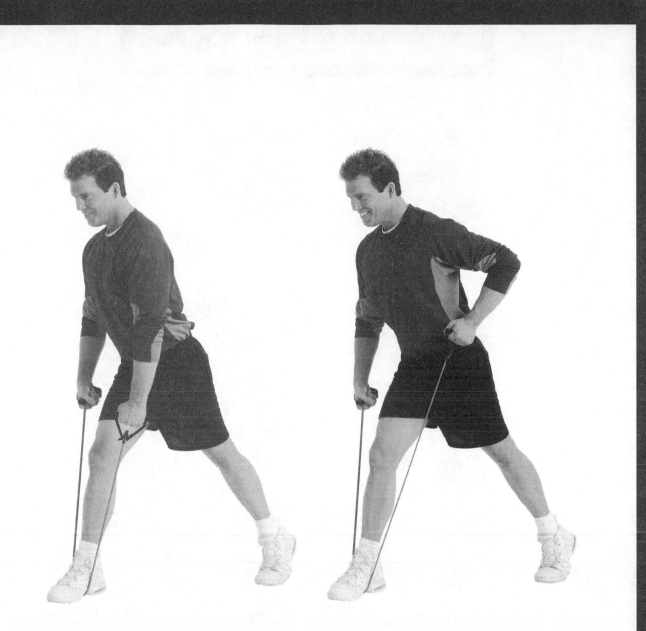

2. SINGLE-ARM TUBING PULL

Target: Back, biceps (elbow flexors), and core

Positioning: Stand with your right foot forward in a slight lunge position with your right foot firmly planted on the floor. The heel of your left foot should be slightly elevated off the floor. Place the tubing securely underneath the arch of your right foot. Hold the short resistance end with your left hand and the slack end in your right hand. Place your upper body at approximately a 45-degree angle to the floor, as shown, and activate your supercenter. Focus downward for optimum neck alignment.

Motion: Draw your left elbow upward so that it just passes your body to form a 90-degree angle at the elbow, as shown. Return to the starting position. Continue the exercise for the recommended number of repetitions, then immediately perform the exercise on the opposite side.

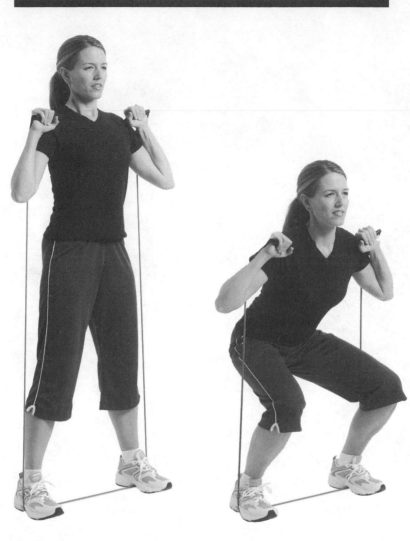

3. TUBING SQUAT PRESS

Target: Quadriceps, hamstrings, glutes (comprehensive lower body), and core

Positioning: Begin with your feet slightly wider than shoulder width apart. Place the tubing underneath the arches of your feet. Hold the handles close in front of the shoulders, as shown. Keep your elbows directly beside your body. In addition, keep your shoulders back and activate your supercenter. Look straight ahead. Your feet stay planted on the floor throughout the exercise.

Motion: Bend your knees to a comfortable range of motion (not past 90 degrees). Keep the entire soles of both feet planted firmly, especially the heels. Make sure that both knees track directly in line between your first and second toes. Press up and return to starting position. Take your time on the downward phase of this motion. Continue the exercise for the recommended number of repetitions.

Tip: If the tubing feels awkward at first, you can perform the exercise with no tubing to start and then add the tubing when you become comfortable with the motion.

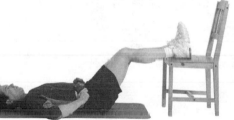

Tip. For added resistance, place a dumbbell or weight plate on your pelvic area, securing it with both hands, as shown.

4. CHAIR BRIDGE (PRESSING MOTION)

Target: glutes and hamstrings (hip and thigh areas)

Positioning: Lie flat on your back. Place the backs of your feet and ankles on a chair or bench, with your knees bent, as shown. Rest your arms at your sides.

Motion: Lift your hips and pelvic area up and toward your face while driving the backs of your feet into the chair or bench. Your rear end will come up off the floor. Raise the hips and pelvic area as high as you can, but do *not* exceed the range of motion shown. Lower toward the starting position, stopping just before your rear end hits the floor, and continue the exercise for the recommended number of repetitions.

5. SUPERMAN (CORE)

Target: Spinal erectors, low back, and glutes

Positioning: Lie facedown on a mat with your arms fully extended overhead and your legs straight. For optimal spinal alignment, keep your face toward the mat. (If this arm position feels uncomfortable in your neck and shoulders, you can place your arms at your sides, as shown in the bottom picture.)

Motion: Lift your arms, your chest, and your legs off of the mat, as shown in the top picture, as though you are flying. Hold this position for 10–15 seconds. Note that you are *holding* this Superman position and not performing the number of reps like you may do in the other exercises. Continue the exercise for the recommended number of static repetitions.

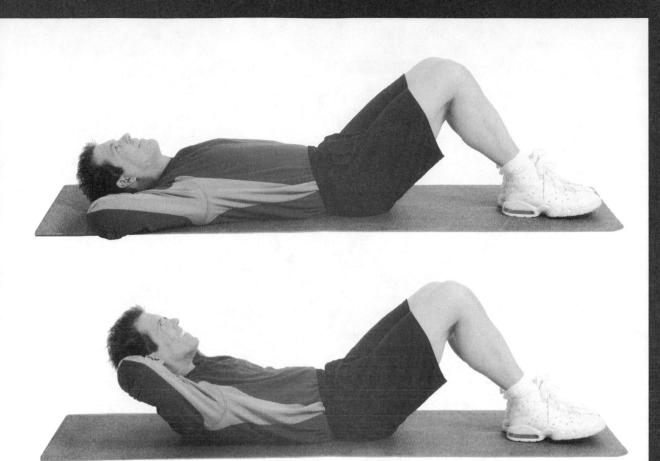

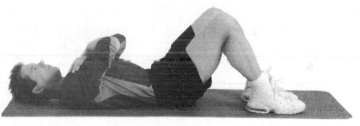

Tip: For added resistance, you can fold your arms across your chest, as shown at right.

6. STANDARD CRUNCH (CORE)

Target: Entire abdominal region

Positioning: Lie on your back on an exercise mat. Bend your knees and place your feet on the floor. Place your hands behind your head for added neck support. Look up at the ceiling to maintain optimal spinal alignment.

Motion: Leading with your chest, raise your upper body toward your knees while keeping your hips stable. Lower and continue the exercise for the recommended number of repetitions. Do not rush this motion, especially on the downward phase.

7. CARDIO BURST

See the directions on page 108-109 for this exercise.

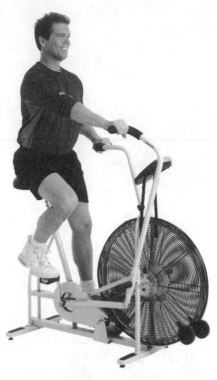

CARDIO BURST
For All Workout Options

Once you've finished your *Make Over Your Metabolism*
resistance training workout, perform a 2-minute "cardio burst"—
a short but maximum intensity all-out effort—in which
you walk fast, jog, run, sprint, bike, jump rope, swim, do
jumping jacks, climb stairs, or use a piece of cardio equipment.
You're already warmed up, so you can absolutely go for it.
Track these daily bursts in your activity journal
so you can see your success!

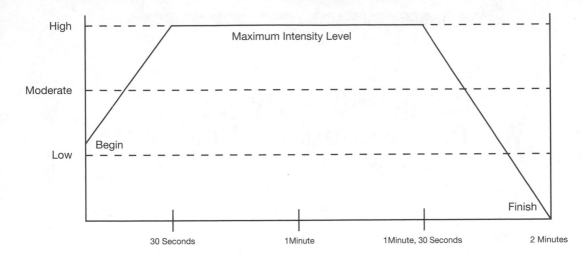

High — — — — — — — — — — — — — — — — — —
Maximum Intensity Level
Moderate — — — — — — — — — — — — — — — — —
Begin
Low — — — — — — — — — — — — — — — — — —
Finish

30 Seconds   1 Minute   1 Minute, 30 Seconds   2 Minutes

YOUR 2-MINUTE "CARDIO BURST"

Here is how to get the most out of your cardio burst: 1. Escalate your pace during the first 30 seconds. 2. Go all out at your *maximum, top-level intensity* for 1 minute. 3. Cool down during the final 30 seconds.

What are the benefits of adding this 2-minute cardio burst to your workout?

•Ensures that you incorporate motion into your day. Remember, our bodies are genetically designed for locomotion. We are meant to move!

•Boosts your metabolism. Even a minimally intense bout of 1–2 minutes can accomplish this, maximizing your workout and postworkout calorie and fat burning.

•Improves your mood by elevating feel-good endorphins in your body.

•Produces positive changes in your cardiorespiratory fitness.

•Energizes you for the day!

*A study done at Colorado State University concluded that 4–5 separate 1-minute bouts of maximum-intensity cardiovascular activity are equal to the total overall caloric expenditure of a 20-minute bout of moderate-intensity activity. Team this with the other bouts of activity during your day such as brisk walks in a parking lot, sprinting to a business meeting, or taking the stairs instead of the elevator.

Tubing and Body-Weight Workout Summary: Beginner

Follow this routine 30 minutes a day, 3 days a week on alternate days. For 3 of the days that you aren't doing the routine, you'll do 30 minutes a day of Metabolic Burst Training (see page 152). The other day is for resting.

*Exercise	Week 1	Week 2	Week 3	Week 4
Standing Tubing Chest Push	2 sets of 10 reps	2–3 sets of 10–12 reps	3 sets of 12 reps	3–4 sets of 10–12 reps
Single-Arm Tubing Pull	2 sets of 10 reps (on each side)	2–3 sets of 10–12 reps (on each side)	3 sets of 12 reps (on each side)	3–4 sets of 10–12 reps (on each side)
Tubing Squat Press	2 sets of 10 reps	2–3 sets of 10–12 reps	3 sets of 12 reps	3–4 sets of 10–12 reps
Chair Bridge	2 sets of 10 reps	2–3 sets of 10–12 reps	3 sets of 12 reps	3–4 sets of 10–12 reps with added resistance**
Superman	2 sets of (static) holds	2–3 sets of (static) holds	3 sets of (static) holds	3–4 sets of (static) holds
Standard Crunch	2 sets of 10 reps	2–3 sets of 10–12 reps	3 sets of 12-15 reps	3–4 sets of 15 reps
Cardio Burst	2 minutes	2 minutes	2 minutes	2 minutes

*Increase the resistance when an exercise begins to feel too easy.
**Add resistance on the Chair Bridge only if you have a weight plate or dumbbell.

My Tubing and Body-Weight Workout

Track your progress each day with this chart. Write in the days you do your resistance training, when you do cardio, and the day you rested. For a more detailed record of your daily activity, make copies of page 254 and fill it in for each day of the program.

	Week 1	Week 2	Week 3	Week 4
Monday				
Tuesday				
Wednesday				
Thursday				
Friday				
Saturday				
Sunday				

Did you meet your goals for each week? In the space below, list any challenges you had for that week and any additional goals you would like to achieve in the following week.

Week 1

Week 2

Week 3

Week 4

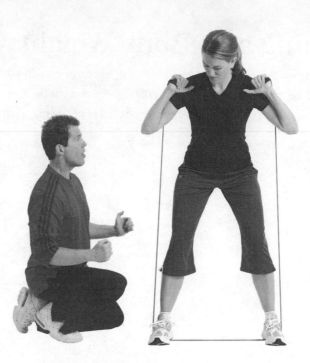

ADVANCED
Tubing and Body-Weight Workout

Once you've completed the first 4 weeks of the Tubing and Body-Weight Workout, you can move up to this advanced option for greater challenges. Follow this routine 3 days a week for the next 4 weeks, again alternating the plan with 3 days of Metabolic Burst Training. Or see page 156 for alternative sequences for your Metabolic Burst Training.

WARM-UP
•4–5 minutes on cardio equipment of choice, marching in place, or walking around •10 seconds of arm circles to the front; 10 seconds of arm circles to the back •12 high knee lifts (alternate 6 per side)

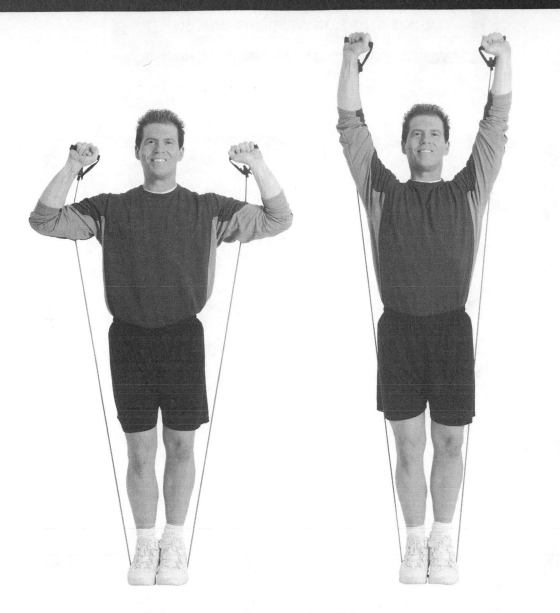

1. STANDING TUBING OVERHEAD PUSH

Target: Shoulders, triceps, balance, and core

Positioning: Stand nice and tall with your feet firmly planted on the floor and your knees slightly bent. Place the tubing directly beneath the arches of both feet or beneath the arch of one foot for less resistance. Grasp the tubing close to your shoulders, as shown. Activate your supercenter so as to not let your lower back arch excessively. Look straight ahead to slightly upward.

Motion: Extend your arms up over your head with the tubing handles in your hands, as shown. Your arm position on full extension overhead should be just slightly in front of your ears. Lower the tubing by bending your arms. Continue for the recommended number of repetitions.

Tip: **If this exercise presents pain or discomfort in your back, neck, or shoulder area, you may substitute the Standing Tubing Lateral Raises (see page 114).**

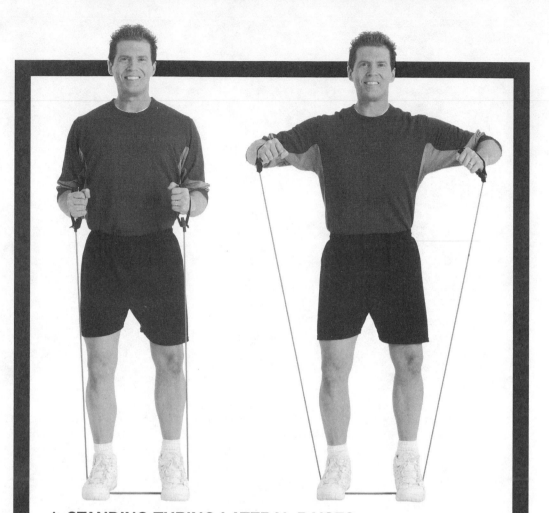

1. STANDING TUBING LATERAL RAISES
(ALTERNATIVE, PUSHING MOTION)

Target: shoulders (front and lateral deltoids)

Positioning: Stand with your feet parallel and approximately shoulder width apart. Keep your knees slightly bent. Activate your supercenter. Place the tubing underneath the middle of both feet (or under one foot only for less resistance). Keep in mind that the closer together your feet are, the *less* resistance you'll feel on this exercise.

Motion: Hold the handles at your sides with your elbows at a 90-degree angle directly beside you. Laterally raise your arms to the side to just below shoulder height, as shown. Return to starting position. Continue the exercise for the recommended number of repetitions.

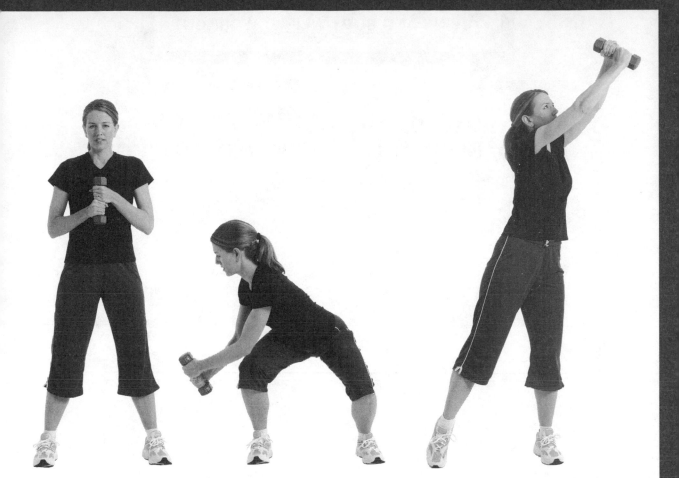

2. LIFE ROTATION (ROTATING AND PRESSING MOTIONS)

Target: Total body, lower body, core, shoulders, and arms

Positioning: Stand nice and tall with your feet firmly planted on the floor, slightly farther than shoulder width apart. Hold a medicine ball or a light dumbbell in front of you. Maintain your supercenter throughout the exercise.

Motion: Bend your knees and squat down, driving your heels into the floor. Rotate your torso to one side (as if picking up a box on the floor beside you). Focus on really using your legs during this exercise. Extend your body back up while lifting the weight or ball across your body and up overhead at a 45-degree angle to the opposite side. Fully extend both arms over to the opposite side as if you were putting this box on a top shelf. Repeat this motion for the recommended amount of reps, then repeat on the other side to complete the set. Note: The listed 12 reps are actually 6 reps to one side immediately followed by 6 reps to the other side, totaling 12 reps for the set.

Tip: You can do this exercise without using either dumbbells or a medicine ball. Add resistance at the appropriate time for you.

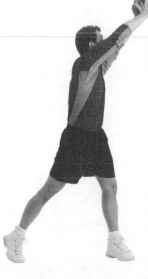

Medicine ball option

115

Tubing and Body-Weight Workout Summary: Advanced

Follow this routine 30 minutes a day, 3 days a week on alternate days. You may continue to perform your Metabolic Burst Training on alternate days from your resistance training. Or check pages 156-157 for alternate scheduling options.

*Exercise	Week 5	Week 6	Week 7	Week 8
Standing Tubing Chest Push	3–4 sets of 10–12 reps	3–4 sets of 10–12 reps	3–4 sets of 12 reps	4 sets of 12 reps
Single-Arm Tubing Pull	3–4 sets of 10–12 reps (on each side)	3–4 sets of 10–12 reps (on each side)	3–4 sets of 12 reps (on each side)	4 sets of 12 reps (on each side)
Tubing Squat Press	3–4 sets of 10–12 reps	4 sets of 10 reps	4 sets of 10 reps	4–5 sets of 12 reps
Chair Bridge	3–4 sets of 10–12 reps	4 sets of 10 reps	4 sets of 10 reps	4–5 sets of 12 reps
Superman	3 sets of (static) holds	3 sets of (static) holds	3 sets of (static) holds	4 sets of (static) holds
Standard Crunch	3–4 sets of 15 reps	3-4 sets of 15 reps	3–4 sets of 15 reps	4 sets of 15 reps
Standing Tubing Overhead Push or Standing Tubing Lateral Raises	2 sets of 10 reps	2 sets of 10 reps	2–3 sets of 12 reps	2–3 sets of 12 reps
**Life Rotation	2 sets of 12 reps	2 sets of 12 reps	2–3 sets of 12 reps	2–3 sets of 12 reps
Cardio Burst	2 minutes	2 minutes	2 minutes	2 minutes

*Increase the resistance when the exercise begins to feel too easy.

**12 reps of Life Rotation are actually 6 reps to each side to complete 1 set.

My Tubing and Body-Weight Workout

Track your progress each day with this chart. Write in the days you do your resistance training, when you do cardio, and the day you rested. For a more detailed record of your daily activity, make copies of page 254 and fill it in for each day of the program.

	Week 5	Week 6	Week 7	Week 8
Monday				
Tuesday				
Wednesday				
Thursday				
Friday				
Saturday				
Sunday				

Did you meet your goals for each week? In the space below, list any challenges you had for that week and any additional goals you would like to achieve in the following week.

Week 5

Week 6

Week 7

Week 8

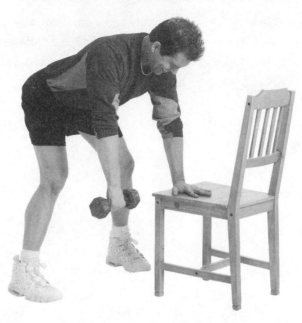

BEGINNER
Chair and Dumbbell Workout

If you prefer using free weights in your workout, the Chair and Dumbbell Workout is a good choice for you. You can pick weights that are appropriate for your level of fitness. As you get stronger you may want to move to a heavier weight. You'll also need a sturdy chair, like the one shown, with solid legs and no cushioning or slippery fabric.

WARM-UP

•4–5 minutes on cardio equipment of choice, marching in place, or walking around •10 seconds of arm circles to the front; 10 seconds of arm circles to the back •12 high knee lifts (alternate 6 per side)

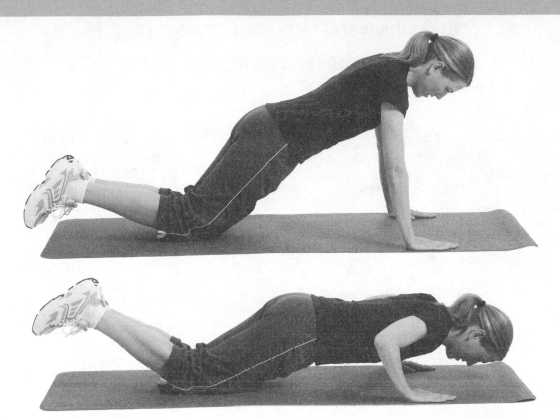

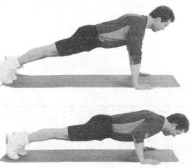

Tip: There actually are three variations of the push-up you can do: the Wall Push-Up that you did in the assessment on page 72; the Knee Push-Up, shown above; or the Standard Push-Up, shown right. Perform the one that is most comfortable yet challenging for you at this point.

1. KNEE PUSH-UP

Target: chest, shoulders, triceps, and core

Positioning: Kneel down and place your palms flat on the floor, directly in line below your shoulder joints, as shown. (You may want to place a towel or pillow underneath your knees to prevent discomfort.) Draw your belly button into your spine, activating your supercenter. Keep your body in one straight line; do not let your back arch excessively or let your body waver. For optimum neck alignment, keep your face down.

Motion: Bend your arms to no more than a 90-degree angle, lowering your chest nearly to the floor. Do not arch your back excessively during the motion. Straighten your arms as you push your upper body up away from the floor. Keep your palms fixed at the same position and keep your body straight. Try not to bend or arch your upper or lower back as you push up. Continue for the recommended number of repetitions.

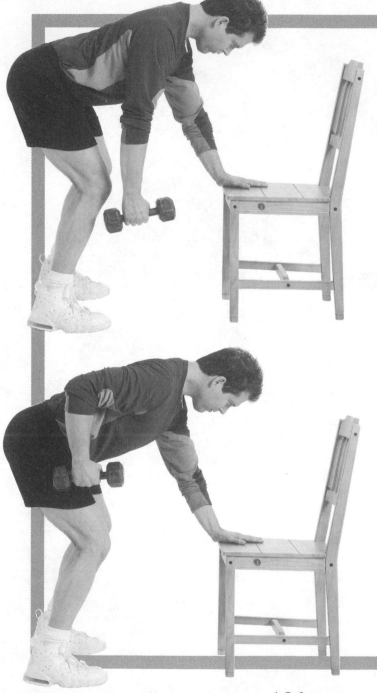

2. SINGLE-ARM DUMBBELL PULL (LOW)

Target: back, biceps (elbow flexors), rear shoulder, and core

Positioning: Begin with your knees slightly bent, with one hand on a chair or bench for added stability. Grasp a dumbbell in the other hand and fully extend your arm toward the floor. Keep your upper body almost parallel to the floor. Look down to assure optimum neck alignment.

Draw your belly button into your spine to activate your supercenter. Keep your body stable throughout the exercise.

Motion: Pull the dumbbell up until your elbow just passes your body. Your arm will form a 90-degree angle at the top of the motion. Extend the dumbbell back down to the starting position. Continue for the recommended number of repetitions and then immediately perform the exercise on the other side.

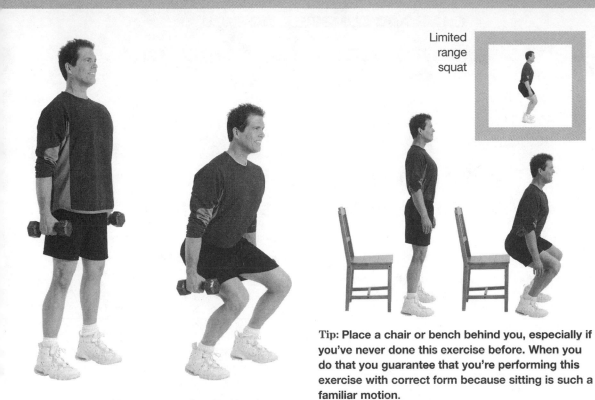

Limited range squat

Tip: Place a chair or bench behind you, especially if you've never done this exercise before. When you do that you guarantee that you're performing this exercise with correct form because sitting is such a familiar motion.

3. BASIC SQUAT PRESS

Target: glutes, hamstrings, quadriceps (comprehensive lower body), and core

Positioning: Stand nice and tall with your feet and heels firmly planted on the floor, slightly farther than shoulder width apart, and your toes pointed to the front. Activate your supercenter by drawing your belly button in toward your spine. Grasp a dumbbell in each hand and hold the weights at your sides. (You may do this exercise with no dumbbells at first, then add the dumbbells when you feel that you are ready for more resistance.) Keep your knees in a "neutral" position—not locked or hyperextended.

Motion: Bend your knees to no more than 90 degrees (go to a comfortable range of motion). Make sure your knees track directly over your toes. Extend your rear end as if you are attempting to sit down on a chair. Descend slowly to maximize every repetition. Return to the standing position. Continue for the recommended number of repetitions.

4. CHAIR BRIDGE (PRESSING MOTION)

See the directions on page 105 for this exercise.

5. SUPERMAN (CORE)

See the directions on page 106 for this exercise.

6. STANDARD CRUNCH (CORE)

See the directions on page 107 for this exercise.

7. CARDIO BURST

See the directions on pages 108–109 for this exercise.

Chair and Dumbbell Workout Summary: Beginner

Follow this routine 30 minutes a day, 3 days a week on alternate days. For 3 of the days that you aren't doing the routine, you'll do 30 minutes a day of Metabolic Burst Training (see page 152). The other day is for resting.

*Exercise	Week 1	Week 2	Week 3	Week 4
Knee Push-Up	2 sets of 10 reps	2–3 sets of 10 to 12 reps	3 sets of 12 reps	3–4 sets of 12 reps
Single-Arm Dumbbell Pull (Low)	2 sets of 10 reps (on each side)	2–3 sets of 10–12 reps (on each side)	3 sets of 12 reps (on each side)	3–4 sets of 10–12 reps (on each side)
Basic Squat Press	2 sets of 10 reps	2–3 sets of 10–12 reps	3 sets of 12 reps	3–4 sets of 10–12 reps
Chair Bridge	2 sets of 10 reps	2–3 sets of 10–12 reps	3 sets of 12 reps	3 sets of 10–12 reps with added resistance
Superman	2 sets of (static) holds	2–3 sets of (static) holds	3 sets of (static) holds	3 sets of (static) holds
Standard Crunch	2 sets of 10 reps	2–3 sets of 10 to 12 reps	3 sets of 12-15 reps	3 sets of 15 reps
Cardio Burst	2 minutes	2 minutes	2 minutes	2 minutes

*Increase the resistance when the exercise begins to feel too easy.

My Chair and Dumbbell Workout

Track your progress each day with this chart. Write in the days you do your resistance training, when you do cardio, and the day you rested. For a more detailed record of your daily activity, make copies of page 254 and fill it in for each day of the program.

	Week 1	Week 2	Week 3	Week 4
Monday				
Tuesday				
Wednesday				
Thursday				
Friday				
Saturday				
Sunday				

Did you meet your goals for each week? In the space below, list any challenges you had for that week and any additional goals you would like to achieve in the following week.

Week 1

Week 2

Week 3

Week 4

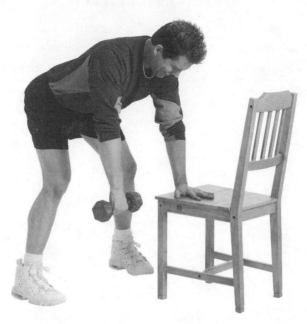

ADVANCED
Chair and Dumbbell Workout

Once you've completed the first 4 weeks of the Chair and Dumbbell Workout, you can move up to this advanced option for greater challenges. Follow this routine 3 days a week for the next 4 weeks, again alternating the plan with 3 days of Metabolic Burst Training. Or see pages 156-157 for alternate sequences for your Metabolic Burst Training.

WARM-UP
•4–5 minutes on cardio equipment of choice, marching in place, or walking around •10 seconds of arm circles to the front; 10 seconds of arm circles to the back •12 high knee lifts (alternate 6 per side)

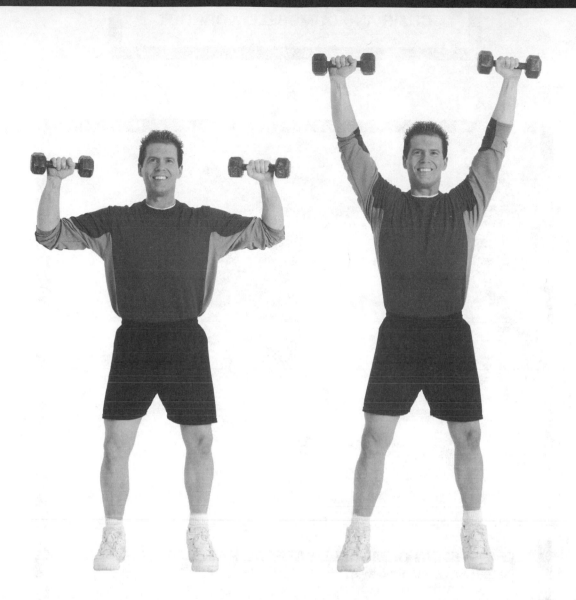

1. STANDING OVERHEAD DUMBBELL PUSH

Target: shoulders, triceps, core, and balance

Positioning: Stand nice and tall with your feet firmly planted on the floor. Activate your supercenter and keep your chest lifted. Look straight ahead to slightly upward. Begin with your elbows bent, holding them to the side and slightly in front of your shoulders. Hold a dumbbell in each hand. Maintain perfect postural and spinal alignment and a comfortable range of motion for your shoulder joints.

Motion: Keeping your elbows to the side and slightly in front of you, extend your arms fully over your head, as shown. Lower the dumbbells slowly to the original position and repeat. Continue for the recommended number of repetitions.

Tip: If this exercise causes pain or discomfort in your back, neck, or shoulder area, you may substitute the Standing Dumbbell Lateral Raise (see page 126).

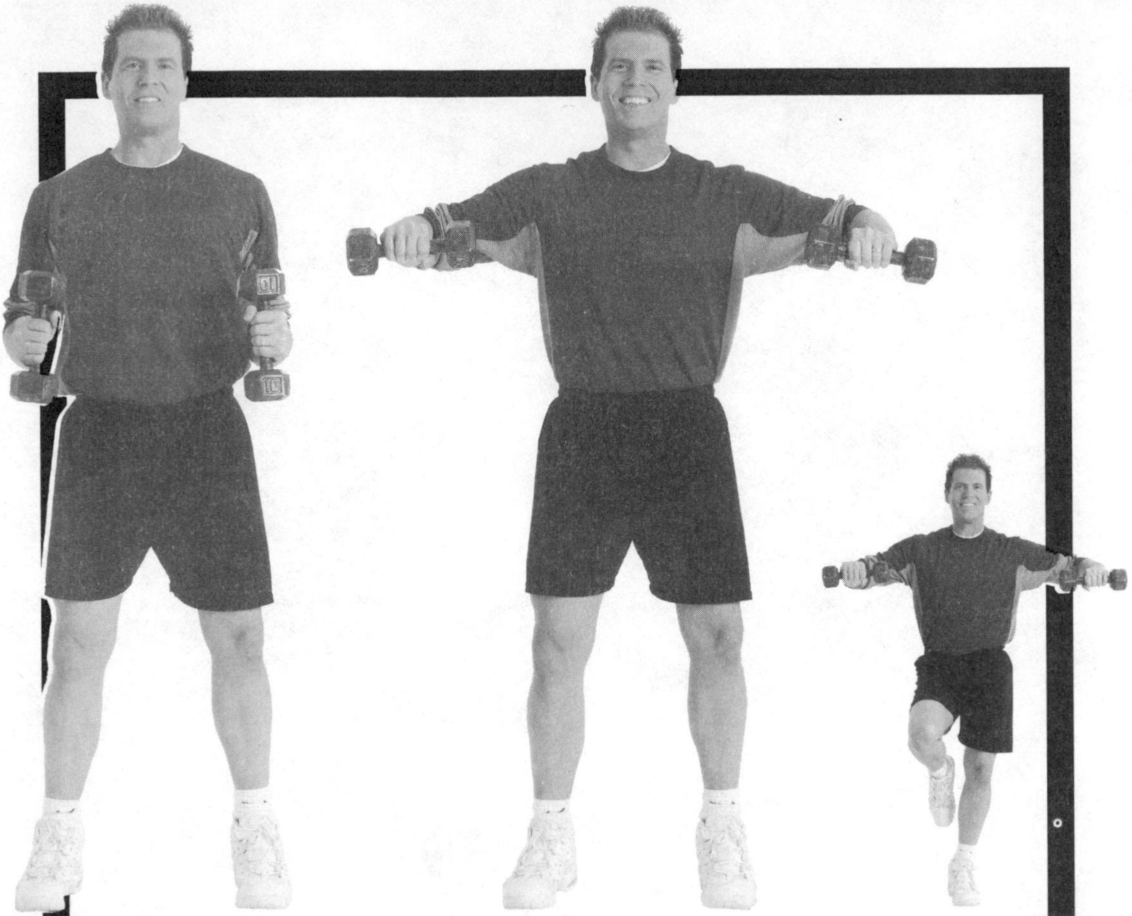

1. STANDING DUMBBELL LATERAL RAISE
(ALTERNATIVE, PUSHING MOTION)
Target: Shoulders, core, and balance

Positioning: Stand nice and tall with your feet firmly planted on the floor. Activate your supercenter and keep your chest lifted. Look straight ahead. Bend your knees slightly. Hold a dumbbell in each hand at your sides with your arms at approximately a 90-degree angle. Maintain perfect posture and spinal alignment and a comfortable range of motion for your shoulder joints.

Motion: Raise your arms directly up from your sides, as shown, to almost shoulder height. Maintain this angle at your elbow joints throughout the motion. Return to starting position and continue the exercise for the recommended number of repetitions.

Tip: For an added challenge, you may perform this exercise while balancing on one foot, as shown above.

126

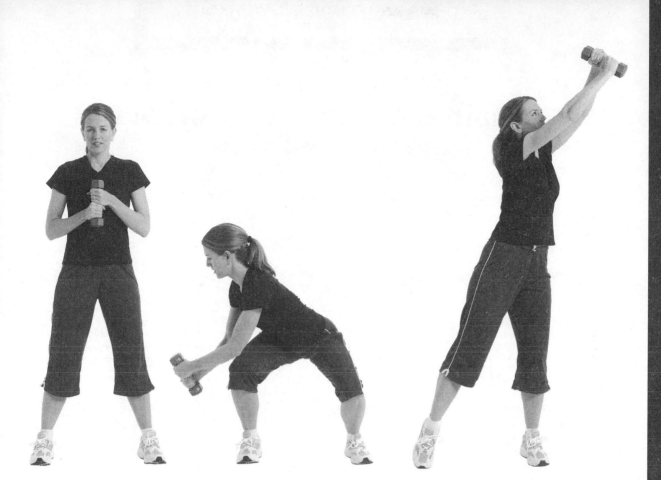

2. LIFE ROTATION (ROTATING AND PRESSING MOTIONS)

See the directions on page 115 for this exercise, which is pictured on this page.

Medicine ball option

Chair and Dumbbell Workout Summary: Advanced

Follow this routine 30 minutes a day, 3 days a week on alternate days. You may continue to perform your Metabolic Burst Training on alternate days from your resistance training. Or check pages 156-157 for alternate scheduling options.

*Exercise	Week 5	Week 6	Week 7	Week 8
Knee Push-Up	3–4 sets of 12 reps	3–4 sets of 10–12 reps	3–4 sets of 10–12 reps	4 sets of 10–12 reps
Single-Arm Dumbbell Pull (Low)	3–4 sets of 10–12 reps (on each side)	3–4 sets of 10–12 reps (on each side)	3–4 sets of 10–12 reps (on each side)	4 sets of 10–12 reps (on each side)
Basic Squat Press	3–4 sets of 10–12 reps	4 sets of 10–12 reps	4 sets of 10–12 reps	4–5 sets of 10–12 reps
Chair Bridge	3–4 sets of 10–12 reps	4 sets of 10–12 reps	4 sets of 10–12 reps	4–5 sets of 10–12 reps
Superman	3–4 sets of (static) holds	3–4 sets of (static) holds	3–4 sets of (static) holds	4 sets of (static) holds
Standard Crunch	3–4 sets of 15 reps	3–4 sets of 15 reps	3–4 sets of 15 reps	4 sets of 15 reps
Standing Overhead Dumbbell Push or Dumbbell Lateral Raise	2 sets of 10 reps	2 sets of 10 reps	2–3 sets of 12 reps	2–3 sets of 12 reps
**Life Rotation	2 sets of 12 reps	2 sets of 12 reps	2–3 sets of 12 reps	2–3 sets of 12 reps
Cardio Burst	2 minutes	2 minutes	2 minutes	2 minutes

*Increase the resistance when the exercise begins to feel too easy.

**12 reps of Life Rotation are actually 6 reps to each side to complete 1 set.

My Chair and Dumbbell Workout

Track your progress each day with this chart. Write in the days you do your resistance training, when you do cardio, and the day you rested. For a more detailed record of your daily activity, make copies of page 254 and fill it in for each day of the program.

	Week 5	Week 6	Week 7	Week 8
Monday				
Tuesday				
Wednesday				
Thursday				
Friday				
Saturday				
Sunday				

Did you meet your goals for each week? In the spaces below, list any challenges you had for that week and any additional goals you would like to achieve in the following week.

Week 5

_____

Week 6

_____

Week 7

_____

Week 8

_____

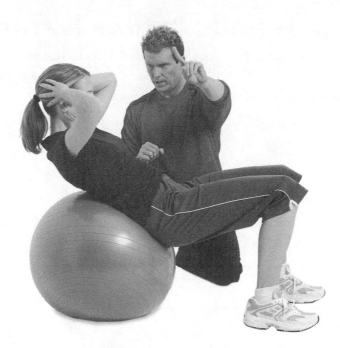

BEGINNER
Stability Ball and Dumbbell Workout

Stability balls are popular because they are inexpensive and easy to use in a variety of workouts. Check out the tips on the next page to make sure you're using the ball safely and correctly. When choosing dumbbells, pick ones that are appropriate for your level of fitness and strength.

WARM-UP
•4–5 minutes on cardio equipment of choice, marching in place, or walking around •10 seconds of arm circles to the front; 10 seconds of arm circles to the back •12 high knee lifts (alternate 6 per side)

ROBERT'S RULES FOR STABILITY BALL SAFETY

• Keep the ball away from young children.

• Only one person at a time should be using the ball during a given exercise.

• Work in an open space free from furniture or other obstacles that may cause injury.

• Use a comfortable and reasonable level of resistance while training with the ball. Do not lift "heavy" weights on the ball.

• Do not exercise in bare feet or socks. Wear proper footwear for maximum stability, balance, and correct motion.

• Keep your eyes open during all exercises.

• Perform all exercises slowly, with control and proper form.

• Do not bounce on the ball.

• Check the floor surface. Do not use the ball on slippery or unstable surfaces.

• Double-check the ball before each workout for any cuts, scratches, worn spots, or other defects. Make sure that the ball is kept away from any sharp or pointed objects. Do not wear jewelry, rings, or other accessories that could puncture or damage the ball.

• Use the correct size ball for your height. (See page 77.)

• Do not abuse the ball by punching or kicking it.

• Avoid using the ball outdoors.

• Store the ball in a safe place and avoid any exposure to sunlight or water.

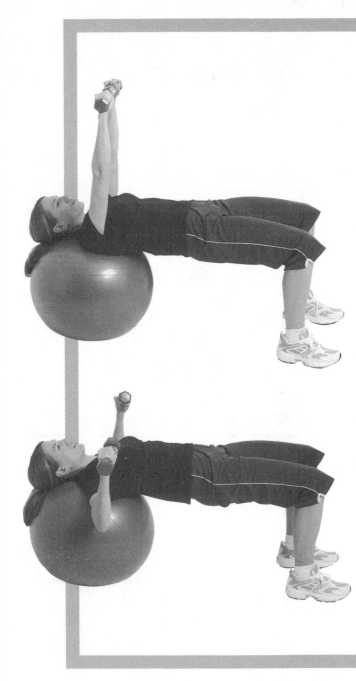

1. BALL CHEST PUSH

Target: chest, shoulders, triceps, core, glutes, quadriceps, hamstrings, and total body stabilization

Positioning: Place the stability ball at the back of your upper shoulders and neck in order to provide comfort for the neck region. Lift your hips until your upper legs are parallel to the floor. Firmly plant your feet on the floor and make sure your knees are directly over your ankles. Maintain this position, as shown, to stabilize your body and work the hip musculature. Hold a dumbbell in each hand. Fully extend your arms so they are perpendicular to the floor.

Motion: Bend your elbows to 90 degrees. Bring your elbows down just slightly below your shoulders. Then press the dumbbells back to the starting position. Continue the exercise for the recommended number of repetitions. By performing this chest press on the ball, you work your target muscles while integrating the rest of your body to provide stabilization. Thus more work is done and more muscle is accessed.

Tip: I recommend practicing this exercise with no dumbbells at first, then adding dumbbells when you feel comfortable with the motion.

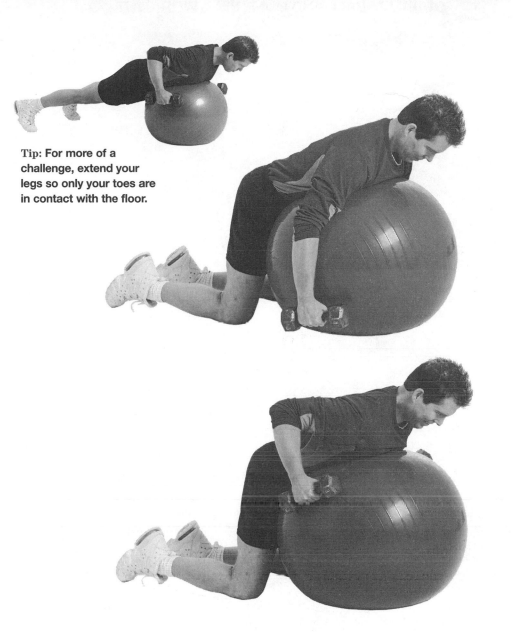

Tip: For more of a challenge, extend your legs so only your toes are in contact with the floor.

2. BALL PULL
Target: back, rear shoulder area, biceps (elbow flexors), core, and total body stabilization
Positioning: Lie over the ball at chest level with your knees on the floor. Grasp dumbbells in each hand and fully extend your arms down. Face downward to keep your neck in proper alignment.
Motion: Draw your elbows back just past your body. At the top of the exercise, your elbows should be at a 90-degree angle. Slightly squeeze your shoulder blades together at the top of this motion. Lower your arms back to the starting position and continue for the recommended number of repetitions.

133

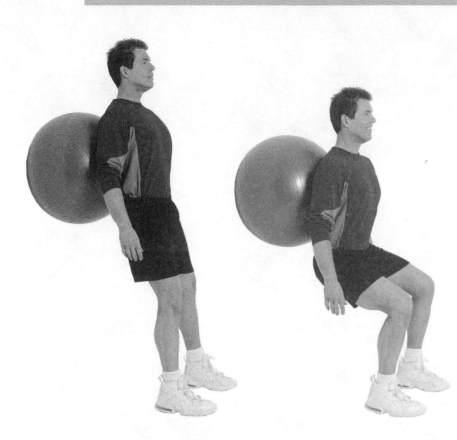

3. BALL WALL SQUAT PRESS
Target: quadriceps, hamstrings, glutes (comprehensive lower body), and core
Positioning: Place the ball against the wall and the back of your body against the ball at around mid-back level, as shown. Stand with your feet planted firmly on the floor a little farther than shoulder width apart. Your toes should face directly forward. Align your knees with your toes. Draw your belly button to your spine while maintaining normal breathing. Keep your chest high and face straight ahead.
Motion: Lower your hips to the floor, using a comfortable range of motion (no more than 90 degrees at the knee). Make sure your knees track with the direction of your toes for optimal and safe knee alignment. Descend slowly to maximize each repetition. Press back up, returning to the starting position. Continue for the recommended number of repetitions.
Tip: For added resistance, hold a dumbbell in each hand.

4. CHAIR BRIDGE (PRESSING MOTION)
See the directions on page 105 for this exercise.

5. SUPERMAN (CORE)
See the directions on page 106 for this exercise.

134

6. BALL CRUNCH WITH ROTATION (CORE)

Target: entire abdominal region

Positioning: Lie faceup on the ball with the ball placed at the mid- to low back area. Plant your feel firmly on the floor. Place your hands behind your head, as shown. Make sure that your upper legs are parallel to the floor.

Motion: Bring your left shoulder/chest area toward your right knee in a rotational motion while keeping your hips and lower body stable. Return to the starting position and repeat the exercise to the opposite side. Alternate the exercise side to side for the recommended number of repetitions.

7. CARDIO BURST

See the directions on pages 108–109 for this exercise.

135

Stability Ball and Dumbbell Workout Summary: Beginner

Follow this routine 30 minutes a day, 3 days a week on alternate days. For 3 of the days that you aren't doing the routine, you'll do 30 minutes a day of Metabolic Burst Training (see page 152). The other day is for resting.

Exercise*	Week 1	Week 2	Week 3	Week 4
Ball Chest Push	2 sets of 10 reps	2–3 sets of 10–12 reps	3 sets of 12 reps	3–4 sets of 10–12 reps
Ball Pull	2 sets of 10 reps	2–3 sets of 10–12 reps	3 sets of 12 reps	3–4 sets of 10–12 reps
Ball Wall Squat Press	2 sets of 10 reps	2–3 sets of 10–12 reps	3 sets of 12 reps	3–4 sets of 10–12 reps
Chair Bridge	2 sets of 10 reps	2–3 sets of 10–12 reps	3 sets of 12 reps	3–4 sets of 10–12 reps
Superman	2 sets of (static) holds	2–3 sets of (static) holds	3 sets of (static) holds	3–4 sets of (static) holds
Ball Crunch with Rotation	2 sets of 10 reps	2–3 sets of 10–12 reps	3 sets of 12-16 reps	3–4 sets of 16 reps
Cardio Burst	2 minutes	2 minutes	2 minutes	2 minutes

*Increase the resistance when the exercise begins to feel too easy.

My Stability Ball and Dumbbell Workout

Track your progress each day with this chart. Write in the days you do your resistance training, when you do cardio, and the day you rested. For a more detailed record of your daily activity, make copies of page 254 and fill it in for each day of the program.

	Week 1	Week 2	Week 3	Week 4
Monday				
Tuesday				
Wednesday				
Thursday				
Friday				
Saturday				
Sunday				

Did you meet your goals for each week? In the space below, list any challenges you had for that week and any additional goals you would like to achieve in the following week.

Week 1

Week 2

Week 3

Week 4

Stability Ball and Dumbbell Workout Summary: Advanced

Follow this routine 30 minutes a day, 3 days a week on alternate days. You may continue to perform your Metabolic Burst Training on alternate days from your resistance training. Or check pages 156-157 for alternate scheduling options.

Exercise*	Week 5	Week 6	Week 7	Week 8
Ball Chest Push (p.132)	3–4 sets of 10–12 reps	3–4 sets of 10–12 reps	3–4 sets of 12 reps	4 sets of 12 reps
Ball Pull (p.133)	3–4 sets of 10–12 reps	3–4 sets of 10–12 reps	3–4 sets of 12 reps	4 sets of 12 reps
Ball Wall Squat Press (p.134)	3–4 sets of 10–12 reps	4 sets of 10 reps	4 sets of 10–12 reps	4–5 sets of 12 reps
Chair Bridge (p.105)	3–4 sets of 10–12 reps	4 sets of 10–12 reps	4 sets of 10–12 reps	4–5 sets of 12 reps
Superman (p.106)	3–4 sets of 3 (static) holds	3-4 sets of 3 (static) holds	3–4 sets of 3 (static) holds	4 sets of 3 (static) holds
Ball Crunch with Rotation (p.135)	3–4 sets of 16 reps	3-4 sets of 16 reps	3–4 sets of 16 reps	4 sets of 16 reps
Overhead Dumbbell Push (p.125) or Lateral Raise (p.126)	2 sets of 10 reps	2 sets of 10 reps	2–3 sets of 12 reps	2–3 sets of 12 reps
Life Rotation** (p.115)	2 sets of 12 reps	2 sets of 12 reps	2 sets of 12 reps	2–3 sets of 12 reps
Cardio Burst (p. 108–109)	2 minutes	2 minutes	2 minutes	2 minutes

*Increase the resistance when the exercise begins to feel too easy.

**12 reps of Life Rotation are actually 6 reps to each side to complete 1 set.

138

My Stability Ball and Dumbbell Workout

Track your progress each day with this chart. Write in the days you do your resistance training, when you do cardio, and the day you rested. For a more detailed record of your daily activity, make copies of page 254 and fill it in for each day of the program.

	Week 5	Week 6	Week 7	Week 8
Monday				
Tuesday				
Wednesday				
Thursday				
Friday				
Saturday				
Sunday				

Did you meet your goals for each week? In the space below, list any challenges you had for that week and any additional goals you would like to achieve in the following week.

Week 5

Week 6

Week 7

Week 8

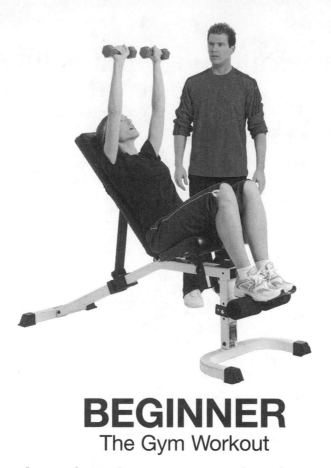

BEGINNER
The Gym Workout

Some people prefer going to a gym rather than working out at
home. If that's you, this is the routine you'll want to follow.
You'll probably want to take the book with you to the gym or
copy the relevant pages and take them with you. If you don't
currently belong to a gym but would like to join, check out my
tips on the next page for finding the gym that's right for you.

WARM-UP
•4–5 minutes on cardio equipment of choice, marching in place, or walking around •10 seconds of arm
circles to the front; 10 seconds of arm circles to the back •12 high knee lifts (alternate 6 per side)

ROBERT'S RULES FOR FINDING A GYM

•Make sure that the gym is conveniently located near your home and/or office. That way you can spend the minimum amount of travel time to and from the facility. If it's out of the way, you're more likely to skip workouts. And optimum convenience and accessibility are major factors that help you stick with your program.

•Make sure that the gym is open at times that fit your schedule.

•Make sure that the gym you want to join makes you feel comfortable.

•Make sure that the facility has the equipment you need for your individual program and goals.

•Make sure that the facility has locker room amenities such as clean showers, bathrooms, and safe storage for your clothes, valuables, and personal items.

•Arrange with either the gym's manager or a qualified trainer to take a tour and get a full orientation on the correct operation of each piece of equipment you will be using. It's necessary that you feel confident and safe when using the equipment.

•Check with the manager of the facility to make sure that all equipment is properly maintained for optimum safety and operation. Report any suspected malfunction immediately to the staff. Be sure to ask about all safety measures that apply specifically to your particular facility.

•Take a towel to every workout unless one is provided for you at the facility.

•Be courteous to all other members working out in the facility. Expect the same courtesy directed toward you from all members and staff.

1. FLAT BENCH DUMBBELL CHEST PUSH

Target: chest, shoulders, and triceps

Positioning: Lie flat on the bench with your feet flat on the bench and your knees up. Keep your body nice and stable. Grasp a dumbbell in each hand and extend your arms straight up, perpendicular to the floor, as shown. Do not lock your elbow joints.

Motion: Slowly lower your arms out to the sides to a position slightly below your shoulders, bending your elbows at a 90-degree angle, as shown. From this position, push the dumbbells back up to the starting position. Continue the exercise for the recommended number of repetitions.

Seated Lat Pulldown

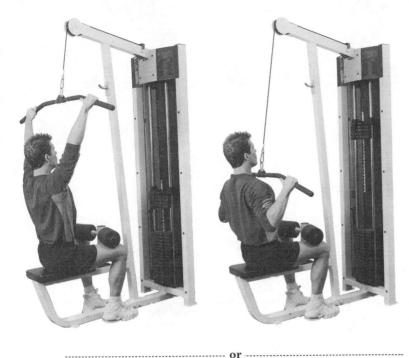

2. SEATED LAT PULLDOWN

Target: back muscles and elbow flexors

Positioning: Sit with your feet planted on the floor and your arms fully extended as you hold the bar around the curved area with your palms facing away from you. Lean back slightly at the waist. Be sure to activate your supercenter.

Motion: Pull your elbows down and in toward your rib cage as your chest meets the bar. Always pull in front of your chest, not behind your neck! In the pulldown position your forearms should be almost perpendicular to the floor. Extend back to beginning position. Continue for the recommended number of reps. Keep your body stable; do not "rock."

-------------------- or --------------------

Seated Row

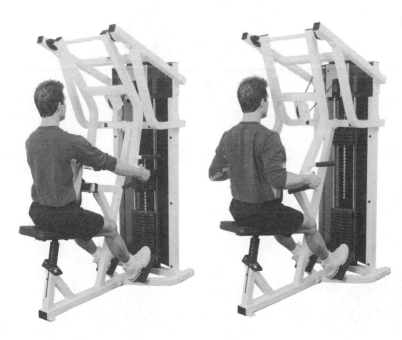

SEATED ROW
(ALTERNATIVE, PULLING MOTION)

Target: back, biceps, rear shoulder, and core

Positioning: Sit up nice and tall on either the seated row machine or a provided platform. Activate your supercenter. Extend your arms straight out in front of you and grasp the handle on the machine, as shown.

Motion: Pull the handle in toward you, drawing your elbows just beyond your torso. At the moment of maximum range of motion, slightly squeeze your shoulder blades together. Straighten your arms back to the original position. Continue for the recommended number of repetitions.

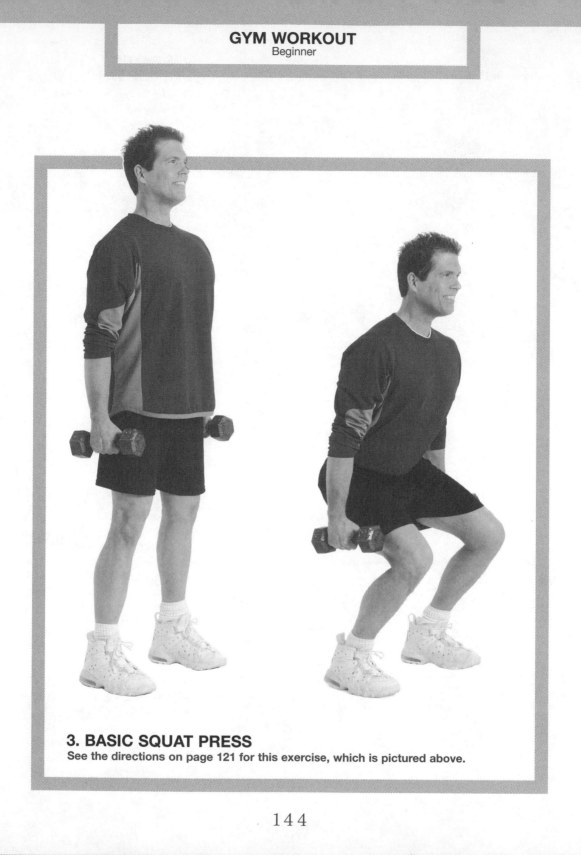

3. BASIC SQUAT PRESS
See the directions on page 121 for this exercise, which is pictured above.

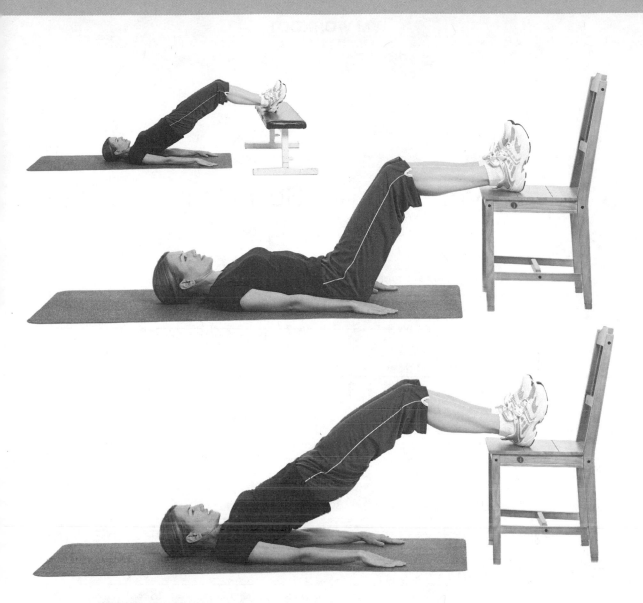

4. CHAIR BRIDGE (PRESSING MOTION)
See the directions on page 105 for this exercise, which is pictured above. You can use either a chair or a bench.

5. SUPERMAN (CORE)
See the directions on page 106 for this exercise.

6. STANDARD CRUNCH (CORE)
See the directions on page 107 for this exercise.

7. CARDIO BURST
See the directions on pages 108–109 for this exercise.

Gym Workout Summary: Beginner

Follow this workout 30 minutes a day, 3 days a week on alternate days. For 3 of the days that you aren't doing the routine, you'll do 30 minutes a day of Metabolic Burst Training (see page 152). The other day is for resting.

Exercise*	Week 1	Week 2	Week 3	Week 4
Flat Bench Dumbbell Chest Push	2 sets of 10 reps	2–3 sets of 10–12 reps	3 sets of 12 reps	3–4 sets of 10–12 reps
Seated Lat Pulldown or Seated Row	2 sets of 10 reps	2–3 sets of 10–12 reps	3 sets of 12 reps	3–4 sets of 10–12 reps
Basic Squat Press	2 sets of 10 reps	2–3 sets of 10–12 reps	3 sets of 12 reps	3–4 sets of 10–12 reps
Chair Bridge	2 sets of 10 reps	2–3 sets of 10–12 reps	3 sets of 12 reps	3–4 sets of 10–12 reps
Superman	2 sets of (static) holds	2–3 sets of (static) holds	3 sets of (static) holds	3–4 sets of (static) holds
Standard Crunch	2 sets of 10 reps	2–3 sets of 10–12 reps	3 sets of 12-15 reps	3–4 sets of 15 reps
Cardio Burst	2 minutes	2 minutes	2 minutes	2 minutes

*Increase the resistance when the exercise begins to feel too easy.

My Gym Workout

Track your progress each day with this chart. Write in the days you do your resistance training, when you do cardio, and the day you rested. For a more detailed record of your daily activity, make copies of page 254 and fill it in for each day of the program.

	Week 1	Week 2	Week 3	Week 4
Monday				
Tuesday				
Wednesday				
Thursday				
Friday				
Saturday				
Sunday				

Did you meet your goals for each week? In the space below, list any challenges you had for that week and any additional goals you would like to achieve in the following week.

Week 1

Week 2

Week 3

Week 4

Gym Workout Summary: Advanced

Follow this routine 30 minutes a day, 3 days a week on alternate days. You may continue to perform your Metabolic Burst Training on alternate days from your resistance training. Or check pages 156-157 for alternate scheduling options.

Exercise*	Week 5	Week 6	Week 7	Week 8
Flat Bench Dumbbell Chest Push (p.142)	3–4 sets of 10 reps	3–4 sets of 10–12 reps	3–4 sets of 12 reps	4 sets of 12 reps
Seated Lat Pulldown or Seated Row (p.143)	3–4 sets of 10 reps	3–4 sets of 10–12 reps	3–4 sets of 12 reps	4 sets of 12 reps
Basic Squat Press (p.121)	3–4 sets of 10 reps	4 sets of 10 reps	4 sets of 10–12 reps	4–5 sets of 10 reps
Chair Bridge (p.105)	3–4 sets of 10–12 reps	4 sets of 10 reps	4 sets of 10–12 reps	4–5 sets of 12 reps
Superman (p.106)	3–4 sets of (static) holds	3–4 sets of (static) holds	3–4 sets of (static) holds	4 sets of (static) holds
Standard Crunch (p.107)	3–4 sets of 15 reps	3–4 sets of 15 reps	3–4 sets of 15 reps	4 sets of 15 reps
Standing Overhead Dumbbell Push (p.125) or Lateral Raise (p.126)	2 sets of 10 reps	2 sets of 10 reps	2–3 sets of 12 reps	2–3 sets of 12 reps
Life Rotation** (p.115)	2 sets of 12 reps	2 sets of 12 reps	2–3 sets of 12 reps	2–3 sets of 12 reps
Cardio Burst	2 minutes	2 minutes	2 minutes	2 minutes

*Increase the resistance when the exercise begins to feel too easy.

**12 reps of Life Rotation are actually 6 reps to each side to complete 1 set.

My Gym Workout

Track your progress each day with this chart. Write in the days you do your resistance training, when you do cardio, and the day you rested. For a more detailed record of your daily activity, make copies of page 254 and fill it in for each day of the program.

	Week 5	Week 6	Week 7	Week 8
Monday				
Tuesday				
Wednesday				
Thursday				
Friday				
Saturday				
Sunday				

Did you meet your goals for each week? In the space below, list any challenges you had for that week and any additional goals you would like to achieve in the following week.

Week 5

Week 6

Week 7

Week 8

COOLDOWN: THE CALMING STRETCH ROUTINE

Every workout should conclude with stretching. This is a very important part of the *Make Over Your Metabolism* program. First, it cools your body down to allow your cardiovascular system to return to normal levels. Second, it increases your suppleness and overall flexibility. Third, it helps your muscles avoid soreness that can occur within eight to 24 hours following your workout. Finally, it lowers stress hormones such as cortisol and adrenaline, calms you, and shifts your body into optimum fat-burning mode for the remainder of the day.

ROBERT'S RULES TO STRETCH BY

•Stretching motions should be gradual and gentle, not fast or jerky. •Hold each stretch in a static position for 10–15 seconds. •Never "bounce" during stretches. •Stretch only to the point of comfortably "feeling it." If the stretch is painful, you've gone too far. •Take your time with your stretching routine. Stretching will help your body recover, both physically and mentally.

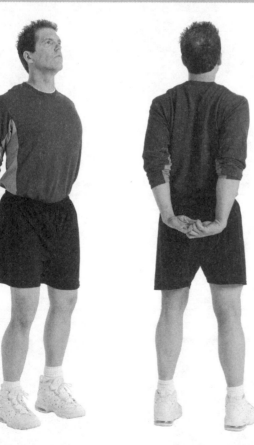

1. STANDING PEC/SHOULDER STRETCH

Target: chest and shoulders

Positioning: Stand nice and tall with your feet firmly planted on the floor and your knees slightly bent.

Motion: Clasp your hands behind you, as shown. Stick your chest out slightly but without letting your low back arch excessively. You should feel this stretch in your chest and shoulder area. Breathe into the stretch.

150

2. STANDING LAT STRETCH

Target: back, lats, and the entire side of the body

Positioning: Stand nice and tall with your feet firmly planted on the floor and your knees slightly bent.

Motion: With one arm, reach directly over to your side and hold, as shown. Repeat on the other side.

3. SEATED HAMSTRING STRETCH

See the directions on page 37 for this exercise.

4. STANDING LIFT AND BREATHE

See the directions on page 34 for this exercise.

Your Metabolic Burst Training
The Initial Four Weeks

Perhaps the most exciting thing about this plan is that you don't have to spend hours and hours on aerobic exercise. This is about the *quality and intensity* of the work, making the most of each and every minute. All this plan requires is 30 minutes of Metabolic Burst Training three times a week. For the initial four weeks, I advise that you perform your Burst Training on days that alternate with your *Make Over Your Metabolism* resistance training workout (3 days of resistance training and 3 days of Metabolic Burst Training). This six-days-per-week approach yields huge daily benefits to your overall metabolism and provides a strong foundation and kick-start to your individual program. For example, if you do your *Make Over Your Metabolism* resistance training workout on Monday, Wednesday, and Friday, perform your Burst Training on Tuesday, Thursday, and Saturday, leaving one day of rest from all exercise. Remember, for your Metabolic Burst Training, all you have to do is alternate short bursts of higher-intensity exercise with moderately paced activity that give your body a little break.

Your 30-Minute Burst Routine for the initial 4-week plan is as follows:

- 4–5 minutes of warm-up (see page 89)
- 20 minutes of 1-minute sprints or "bursts" alternating with 1 minute of lower-intensity "cruise" work (see graph page 91)
- 3–4 minutes of cooldown, followed by 1–2 minutes of the same four calming stretches used in the resistance training.

Keep in mind again that a "sprint" is your high-intensity 1-minute interval. High intensity refers to your top effort—the very best you can do. Try to reach the highest range of your heart rate training zone (see "Heart Rate Monitoring," page 154).

Your "cruise" is your lower- or moderate-intensity 1-minute interval. This minute provides "active rest" to prepare you for the high-level intensity minute to follow. Moderate intensity means your "medium" effort. This is certainly not your highest intensity, but it is definitely not your lowest. This is the midrange of your heart rate training zone.

Low intensity is your basic "beginning" level. This is the lower range of your heart rate training zone and is predominately achieved during "cruise" intervals only.

The intensity level recommendations are for your *individual* intensity levels. For example, your highest level of intensity may be 55 percent of your maximum heart rate. You can always achieve your highest level for a given workout on a given day—after all, it's *your* level and this is *your* program. You will improve over time with consistent commitment to this program, and you will be able to see this improvement in your journal.

Metabolic Burst Training Exercise Options

You have plenty of exercise options for Metabolic Burst Training. Remember, variety is a big factor in keeping you interested in and committed to exercising. It's important that you choose activities that you enjoy and feel comfortable doing. Consider these terrific options for your Metabolic Burst Training "sprints" and "cruises":

- **Fast walking on a treadmill** combined with slower treadmill walking
- **Running outside** combined with slower-paced jogging outside
- **Jumping jacks or walking up stairs** combined with walking in the gym, mall, or outside
- **Power walking outside** combined with jumping rope outside
- **Cycling fast on a stationary bike** combined with cycling slower on a bike
- **Cycling outside on inside at a high resistance** combined with cycling outside at a lower resistance
- **Swimming with an innertube or a kickboard and doing high-intensity leg pumps** alternating with lower-intensity leg pumps
- **Swimming laps at a high-intensity** followed by swimming laps at a lower intensity
- **Using an elliptical trainer at high intensity** and using an elliptical trainer at low or moderate intensity
- **Jumping rope at home** alternating with marching in place
- **Walking up stairs in the mall** combined with walking on a flat area in the mall
- **Dancing to your favorite music at high intensity** and then dancing at a lower intensity
- **Jumping jacks or "step-ups"** (see photo on page 248) and a moderate-intensity walk around the house or office
- **"Air" boxing or hitting a heavy bag at high intensity** and then skipping rope at a moderate pace
- **Rowing on a rowing machine at high intensity** and at a slower pace

You don't need to buy expensive equipment or sign up for special classes. (Although I do recommend classes for physical activity, if this is something you enjoy.) Metabolic Burst Training can be done indoors or outdoors using treadmills, stationary bikes, elliptical trainers, stair-climbing machines, the pavement, a park, a school, the office grounds, the mall, the Deluxe Exerciser (see pages 158-159), or a swimming pool.

You do not need to use the same mode of training every day. Using different exercises in various combinations, there are endless ways you can organize your Metabolic Burst Training workouts. If you vary your workouts, you're less likely to become bored, and your body will show even stronger results. Changing your mode of exercise can keep your body from adapting, so you may even burn more calories. Wear your pedometer so that your workout counts toward your daily step total. The key is to choose the best option for you, including available equipment and venue, and follow it like a road map.

Safety Points for Metabolic Burst Training

Avoid running down steep hills as this can potentially damage your knees. Instead, walk down hills at a comfortable pace so that you have full control of your body.

When walking or running on stairs for exercise, hold on to the rails for balance and always walk down the stairs under full control.

At the beginning you may not be able to complete the recommended 30 minutes of Metabolic Burst Training. This is absolutely OK. Give your best effort and record how much time you did accomplish in your journal, then build from that point. This program is all about achieving your individual best, and as long as you have done your best on a given day, that day is a success.

Heart Rate Monitoring

I strongly recommend using a heart rate monitor when performing Burst Training or lifting weights. This monitor indicates your heartbeats per minute (bpm) and is one of the best ways to evaluate your exercise intensity and track your progress. I recommend the Mio heart rate monitor. It provides ECG accuracy and does not require the use of a chest strap. You'll find that after working out on a regular basis, you can do more work with less effort.

If you do not have a heart rate monitor, you can check your pulse by placing two fingers lightly on your wrist (on the thumb side). Count the heartbeats for 10 seconds, multiply by 6, and you'll find your beats per minute.

Generally speaking, you want to work out at between 55 and 95 percent of your maximum heart rate (MHR). Calculate your appropriate heart rate simply by subtracting your age from 220 and multiplying the result by your desired intensity percentage. For example, the target zone for a 40-year-old exerciser who wants to work at between 65 and 75 percent of her MHR would be 117 to 135 beats per minute.

$$220 - 40 = 180. \quad 180 \times .65 = 117 \text{ BPM.} \quad 180 \times .75 = 135 \text{ BPM.}$$

The closer you can get to 95 percent intensity on your "sprint" intervals, the better, although intensity is relative to your present fitness level and ability on a given day. This is very important to remember as you begin and progress through this program. Again this is about working at your own highest intensity level, whatever level that may be at this time.

Keep in mind that when I say "sprint" I don't necessarily mean an all-out sprint. Instead, I'm asking for your best effort. Your highest intensity at the onset of this pro-

Heart Rate Chart for Men and Women

Age	55%	65%	75%	85%	95%
20	110 bpm	130 bpm	150 bpm	170 bpm	190 bpm
30	105 bpm	124 bpm	143 bpm	162 bpm	181 bpm
40	99 bpm	117 bpm	135 bpm	153 bpm	171 bpm
50	94 bpm	111 bpm	128 bpm	145 bpm	162 bpm
60	88 bpm	104 bpm	120 bpm	136 bpm	152 bpm
70	83 bpm	98 bpm	113 bpm	128 bpm	143 bpm
80	77 bpm	91 bpm	105 bpm	119 bpm	133 bpm

gram may be 50 or 55 percent of your maximum heart rate. Eventually you will achieve higher intensities like 65, 75, 85, and even 95 percent of your maximum heart rate. In other words your individual "training zone" will increase as your fitness level increases. For example, a level of 55 percent may be a challenge today, but one month from now you may need to raise the high-intensity range of your target heart rate "training zone" to 65 percent or higher.

Aim for intensity levels that are comfortable yet challenging, and record your levels in your exercise journal (located in the Appendix) so you can see and acknowledge your daily improvements. Remember, your heart rate will fluctuate during Burst Training because you are alternating bursts with cruises.

Above all, check with your physician about what your high-intensity heart rate should be, based on your present condition and fitness level. The heart rate chart on page 155 will help you find the general range you're after, based on your age.

Your Recovery Heart Rate

An important way to determine if you are reaping the benefits from exercise is to calculate your recovery heart rate, which indicates how quickly you return to your resting heart rate after a workout.

To calculate your recovery heart rate, check your heart rate immediately after you have finished exercising, just before your cooldown stretch. Write the number down in your journal. One minute later, check your heart rate again and write it down. This number is your recovery heart rate.

Monitor your recovery heart rate after each exercise session and keep track of it in your journal. The faster the number drops, the better shape you're in.

Beyond the First Four Weeks

Once you have completed four weeks of Burst Training, feel free to change the sequence and scheduling of your program. Here are some options to consider:

- **Combine the *Make Over Your Metabolism* Resistance Training Workouts and Metabolic Burst Training into a one-hour workout.** Again this approach should be done so that you work out one day and take the next day off. If you go this route, be sure to do your resistance training first (after you warm up, of course). This will optimize the hormonal response that maximizes your body's ability to build fat-burning muscle.

Your "tank" is full of carbohydrate "fuel" when you do resistance training first, giving you the energy you need to derive the most benefit from your resistance work. Also, more body fat is burned overall when you select this sequence.

- **Do the *Make Over Your Metabolism* Resistance Training Workout and Metabolic Burst Training on the same day, but in separate 30-minute workouts.** If you do Metabolic Burst Training in the morning and wish to do your resistance training in the afternoon or early evening, allow a five- to six-hour separation to maximize the muscle building and hormonal response from your resistance workout.

- **Do 30 minutes of your *Make Over Your Metabolism* Resistance Training Workout, then spread Metabolic Burst Training throughout the day.** For example, you may do the 30-minute resistance training during the morning, with Metabolic Burst Training divided into three 10-minute portions or two 15-minute portions spaced throughout the day. In 1995 a group of scientific investigators was formed by the Centers for Disease Control and Prevention and the American College of Sports Medicine to review the pertinent research regarding exactly how much exercise Americans need and how best to get it. This group concluded that every adult in the United States should accumulate a minimum daily caloric expenditure from exercise and that the activity does not need to be continuous. In fact it was stated that the "accumulation of physical activity in intermittent, short bouts is considered an appropriate approach to achieving the activity goal." Activities spread throughout your day provide an excellent added "boost" to your overall metabolism.

- **Squeezing in shorter workouts during the day is an effective way to lose weight and build overall fitness, especially for people with hectic schedules—which is most of us.** You might do 15 minutes of Burst Training before your children wake up in the morning and after they go to bed at night. Or get your first 10-minute burst in before you jump into the shower in the morning. At lunchtime shut your office door and do 10 minutes of jumping jacks, or go outside and walk, or head to the corporate fitness center for 10 minutes. Right before dinner do your final 10-minute burst. So there you have it—30 minutes of Burst Training easily folded into your day.

- **A day of resistance training alternating with a day of Metabolic Burst Training.** As in the initial four-week plan, you'll do your 30-minute resistance training one day, then do the Metabolic Burst Training—which you can break down into smaller portions such as three 10-minute sessions or two 15-minute sessions—on the other days.

A Specialty Program If You Have Special Needs

Over the years working with the *Dr. Phil* show, I have received many e-mails from people crying out for help because they are chair-bound due to injury, illness, orthopedic problems, or profound obesity. They want to start an exercise program—they really do—but they can't even get out of their chairs. They have asked me, "What can I do?"

If you can relate to this situation, I want to address your special needs. Until now no one has probably ever thought of you as an exerciser. Well I think about you, and I have an answer.

It is a device called a Deluxe Exerciser. You can place it on the floor and pedal with your feet while you're sitting in a chair or at your desk. Or you can place it on a desk or

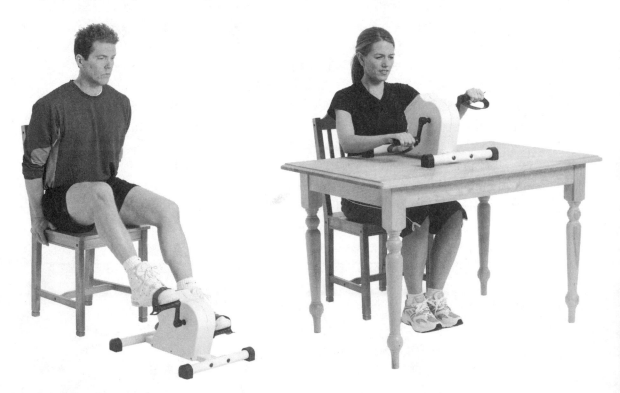

a table and pedal using your arms. As your fitness level improves, you can adjust the resistance on the device to increase the challenge.

Now, how should you use the Deluxe Exerciser? I've designed an easy-to-do specialty program just for you. Four days a week, I'd like you to exercise in the following manner:

- 5-minute pedal with your legs
- 5-minute pedal with your arms
- Perform this sequence twice a day.

The athlete in *you* is ready to come out. You may not be ready for the exercise program I've outline in this chapter, but you want to get going. Be sure to speak to your physician and discuss your plans to include the *Make Over Your Metabolism* program in your life. For information on how to order a Deluxe Exerciser, see the Resources section in the back of this book.

Moving Forward

Congratulations! Whether you have made it through one workout or the eight-week program, you should feel successful—because you are. By the two-week mark, you can expect positive changes to occur in your body. Your muscles will be stronger, so you'll be able to use resistance much more efficiently. Pretty soon the muscles will be harder and more defined. The thermostat on your calorie- and fat-burning furnace will be elevated to new levels. With Metabolic Burst Training in your exercise mix, you'll start to see curves in places you have always wanted them. Your energy level will soar. Every time you train, every time you eat a healthy meal, every time you make a positive choice, every night you get eight hours of sleep, you are becoming the best you can be.

The day will come when your body will want new challenges, however. It will demand a new training effect. That's when you have to incorporate different strategies into your workout to keep stimulating muscle development. These strategies are covered in the next chapter. You'll learn how to take your body to new levels of fitness. Your body fat will continue to drop. Your waist will get trimmer. So will your thighs and hips. You body will become better proportioned. Your personal best will be even better. Sound exciting? Turn the page, and you'll see just how to make it all happen.

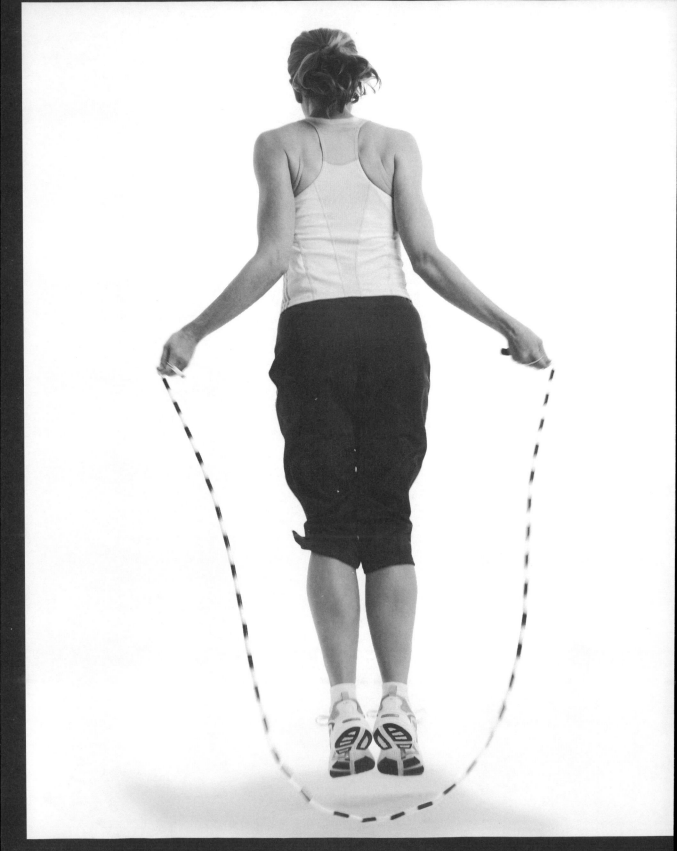

Chapter Seven

W E KIDDINGLY CALL PARTS OF OUR BODY "SADDLEBAGS" OR "LOVE HANDLES" OR "THUNDER THIGHS." REGARDLESS OF THE NICKNAMES, WE ALL HAVE THEM: TROUBLE SPOTS THAT JUST DON'T SEEM TO COME ALONG AS QUICKLY as others or that never quite measure up to our standards. They need some special attention. This chapter will give you some shape-specific advice on how to exercise those parts of your body that you'd like to improve.

First let me clarify something I'm sure you've heard many, many times before: There is no such thing as spot fat reduction. You cannot physically work fat off one specific area of your body at one time. But there is something I call "spot conditioning," and it will make a huge difference in how you look, provided you also follow the Nutritional Life Plan in Chapters 8 and 9.

Spot Conditioning and Staying Active

The physiological truth is that we lose fat wherever we have a genetic predisposition to burn fat, just as we gain more fat in certain areas than we do in others. So if you think fat isn't leaving your thighs fast enough, it's only because that's an area where you store more fat. The great news is that our systems work as a unit to burn fat everywhere on our bodies. So spot conditioning our lower bodies (which is where our largest muscle groups are) will increase the trimming of fat in our thighs as well as our midsections and upper bodies. Although fat burning is a systemic phenomenon that occurs at pretty much an even rate in all areas, you can work the muscles in those areas to maximize your metabolism while giving those muscles shape that results in a trim, tight look and feel. You can use additional training routines and Metabolic Burst Training options (see pages 153 and 203–204) to help get your trouble spots into shape and resculpt your body. This is what my spot-conditioning program is all about.

By combining spot conditioning with the workout options in chapter 6, Metabolic Burst Training, my lifestyle tips, and the Nutritional Life Plan, your body will be strongly coaxed into burning the fat that may be covering your muscles. Yes, you can absolutely accomplish this in three hours a week. But now that you're in better shape and more attuned to exercising, I encourage you to further the progress you've made by occasionally putting in a little more time for shape-specific work, additional Burst Training options, and sports and leisure activities. Keep in mind that as your fitness program keeps progressing over time, you will desire new and different challenges to keep it fun and exciting. The following workouts will help you keep things fresh for a lifetime of fitness. This is in essence an *extension* of the "road map" provided in the rest of this book. If you feel like enhancing your workouts with bonus or alternative specialty exercises, let's get going!

Spot-Conditioning Routines

I have designed five spot-conditioning routines, based on the common "trouble spot" concerns I hear from my clients:

- **Thigh Toner Routine:** Use this workout if you'd like to trim down your thighs and hips while simultaneously enhancing the fat-burning capacity of your entire body. In doing so you will reshape your body to appear less "bottom heavy" and more proportional. There is one Thigh Toner Workout for use at the gym and one for use at home.
- **Ab Tightening Core Routine:** Use this workout to get additional

midsection shaping and firming. I believe everyone has the potential to develop firm abdominals. It takes proper diet, total body resistance training, and Metabolic Burst Training to strip off the fat that surrounds the abs and the right exercises to develop the ab muscles. With that combination everyone can have sexy, attractive abdominals. This workout will help you get there. Keep in mind that there is much more to your midsection than your abs. By activating your supercenter during all of your workouts, you are greatly enhancing both the appearance and function of your entire midsection. So think of this workout as another great opportunity to spot-condition while enhancing your metabolism.

- **Upper-Body Balance Routine:** If you feel you're too muscular in your lower body, these exercises will make your body more proportional since it's focusing on development of your top half. Over the years I've worked with many women, from former competitive athletes to dancers, who have a propensity to build muscle very quickly in their lower bodies. If this describes you, I recommend that you incorporate this specialty workout, as well as some of the Upper-Body Focus Routine exercises (see below) and additional Metabolic Burst Training Workouts. By continuing to develop your upper body while letting the already potent fat-burning machinery in your lower body continue to work for you 24-7, it becomes a matter of getting more aggressive and consistent with your Metabolic Burst Training. Then you are home free to success.

- **Upper-Body Focus Routine:** If you'd like to build your upper body, particularly your pectoral muscles, which give your chest an attractive lift, along with the posture-enhancing muscles of the back, then you'll love this workout. There is a workout option for use at the gym and a workout option for use at home. Both options include "pushing" motions—which focus on the chest, shoulder, and tricep musculature—and "pulling" motions—which focus on the muscles of the back and bicep (elbow flexor) regions.

- **Medicine Ball Routine:** Use this routine if you feel "round all over" and need some extra exercises to reproportion your body to more attractive dimensions. This is a total body workout that I recommend everyone use frequently. This specialty workout takes little time and will enhance your overall balance, strength, stability, and coordination, adding a dramatically effective fat-burning element to the *Make Over Your Metabolism* program.

These spot-conditioning routines may be performed in addition to those routines covered in Chapter 6 or in place of certain exercises in each routine in Chapter 6. Below are some guidelines for incorporating my specialty spot-conditioning routines into the second (advanced) four weeks, as well as for progressing beyond the initial eight weeks.

- **Add the Ab Tightening Core Routine or Medicine Ball Routine** to *any* of the *Make Over Your Metabolism* Workouts from Chapter 6 or perform them on days that you don't do a routine. Incorporating these spot-conditioning routines will continue to elevate your overall fitness level and expand your fat-burning capacity. Note: These two routines should be incorporated during the advanced phase (the second four-week segment) of the *Make Over Your Metabolism* Workouts. You may also incorporate them during the initial four-week routines, if you desire the added workout time.
- **If you prefer to focus on your lower body** to maximize your body's fat-burning capabilities, replace the lower body exercises in any of the Chapter 6 workouts with the Thigh Toner Routine.
- **If you want to streamline your upper body,** replace the upper body exercises in any of the Chapter 6 routines with the Upper-Body Focus Routine.
- **Try split routines.** After completing the first eight weeks of the *Make Over Your Metabolism* program, you may want to amp up your strength training and employ "split routines." This is an ultraintense four-week protocol in which you perform the Thigh Toner Routine on one day and then the Upper-Body Focus Routine on the next. This six-day-per-week strength training regimen will send your fitness and fat-burning capacities soaring! You can toss in the Medicine Ball Routine and Ab Tightening Core Routine two to four times per week as well. And of course remember to keep doing your Metabolic Burst Training. This is clearly an advanced protocol.

Note: With whatever spot-conditioning routine you choose, if you work a particular area of the body, you must wait 36–48 hours before working that area again. The exceptions to this rule are the Medicine Ball Routine and Ab Tightening Core Routine, which can be done on consecutive days.

It's also very important to note that the range of repetitions per set for these spot-conditioning routines is relatively wide compared to the *Make Over Your Metabolism*

Workouts in Chapter 6. The reason is that you now have the knowledge to gear your workouts more specifically to your individual needs. Generally, if your desire is to challenge and build more muscle, you will stay toward the lower rep range with a higher resistance level. If you are not interested in building more muscle but in maintaining and improving the definition you've accomplished thus far, shoot for higher repetitions with less resistance. Over the years my clients have had major success and consistent results at the higher rep ranges—10, 12, and 15 reps per set. You can now customize *your* particular workouts to *your* particular needs, and you now have the road map to do just that.

WARM-UP

• 4–5 minutes on cardio equipment of choice, marching in place, or walking • 10 seconds of arm circles to the front; 10 seconds of arm circles to the back • 12 high knee lifts (alternate 6 per side)

1. BASIC SQUAT PRESS

See directions on page 121 for this exercise.

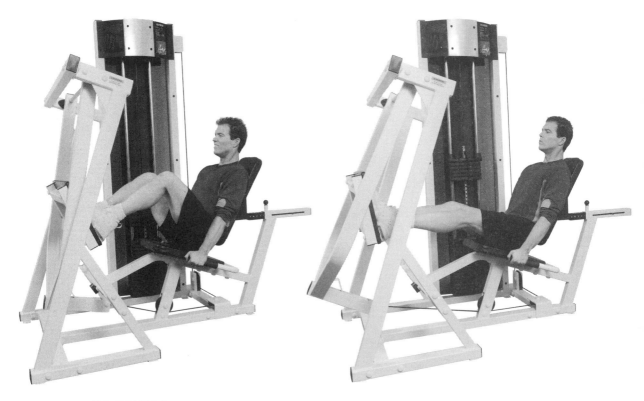

2. LEG PRESS

Target: lower body

Positioning: Sit in the leg press machine with your back against the padded support. Place your feet firmly on the platform and grasp the side handles.

Motion: Push the platform away from you by extending your legs and driving your feet into the platform. On the return phase, bring your knees to no more than a 90-degree angle, then extend your legs back to the original position. Do not let your knees lock. Continue for the recommended number of repetitions.

Tip: You will see many different versions of leg press machines in various facilities. Some will be at a 45-degree angle, others horizontal. Regardless of the machine's design, the basic technique for the exercise remains the same.

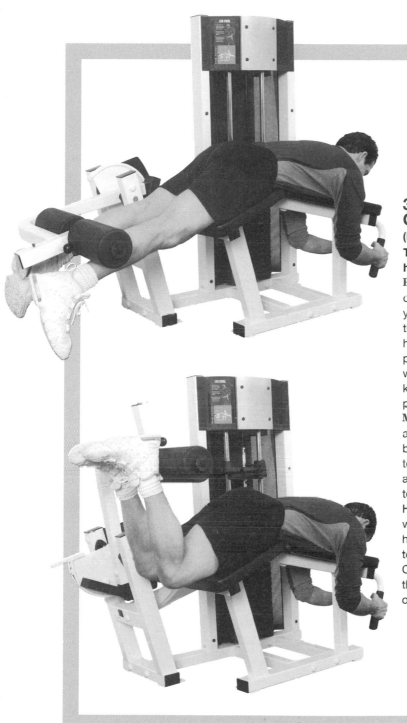

3. HAMSTRING CURLS
(PULLING MOTION)

Target: hamstrings and hip area

Positioning: Lie facedown on a leg curl machine with your knees just below or off the bench and your heels hooked behind the roller pads. Fully extend your legs with a slight bend at your knees. Your toes should be pointing down.

Motion: Keeping your hips and pelvic area against the bench, lift your heels up toward your buttocks in an arc so that your legs bend to about a 90-degree angle. Hold for a brief moment while contracting your hamstring muscles. Return to the original position. Continue the exercise for the recommended number of repetitions.

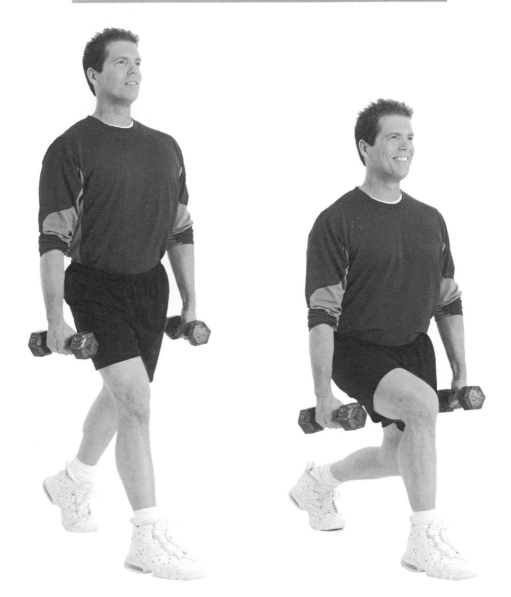

4. STATIONARY DUMBBELL LUNGE (PRESSING MOTION)

Target: Quadriceps, hamstrings, glutes, and total hip area

Positioning: Grasp a dumbbell in each hand and hold the weights at your sides. Begin with your right foot forward, firmly planted about 1–2 feet in front of your left foot. The heel of your left foot should be slightly off the floor. Activate your supercenter. Keep your shoulders back and face straight ahead.

Motion: Bend your right knee to a comfortable range of motion (not past 90 degrees). Return to the original position and continue the exercise for the recommended number of repetitions. Repeat on the opposite leg.

168

5. HEEL RAISES (PRESSING MOTION)

Target: Calf muscles

Positioning: Stand on the edge of a step unit, holding on to a chair for stability, as shown. Keep your knees neutral (not locked) and activate your supercenter.

Motion: Raise your heels as high as they will go, then lower them to just below the surface of the step, maximizing your range of motion. Continue the exercise for the recommended number of repetitions.

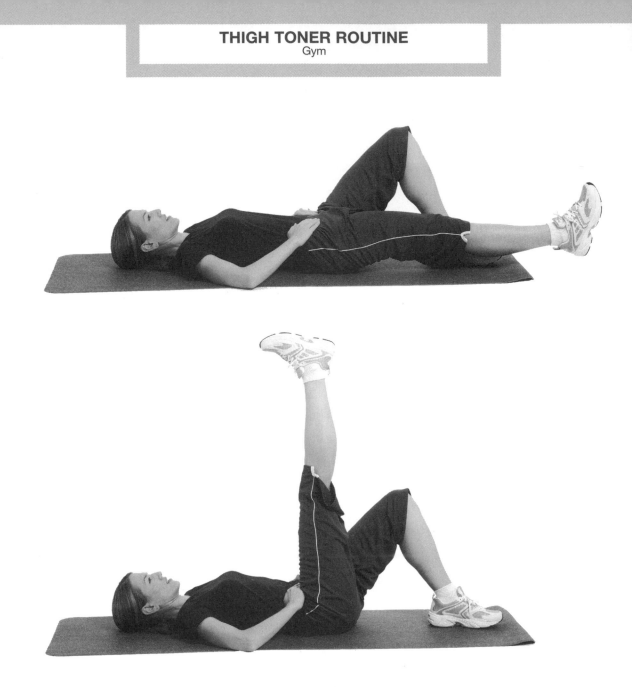

6. STRAIGHT-LEG FRONT LEG LIFTS (PUSHING MOTION)

Target: quadriceps, hip flexors

Positioning: Lie flat on your back with your left knee bent and left foot flat on the floor.

Motion: Keep your right leg straight. Lift it up until it is almost perpendicular to the floor. Lower your right leg until it almost reaches the floor and continue for the recommended number of reps. Repeat the exercise on the opposite leg.

Tip: You can increase the intensity of this exercise by incorporating some ankle weights.

170

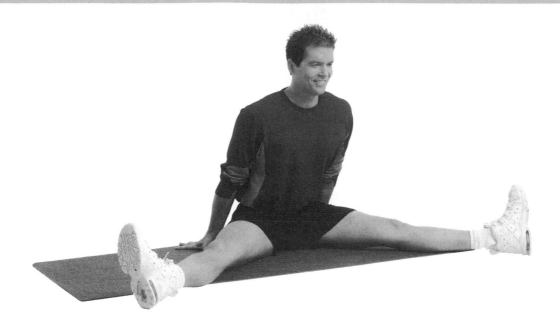

7. FLOOR "V" CENTER STRETCH
See directions on page 44 for this exercise, which is pictured above.

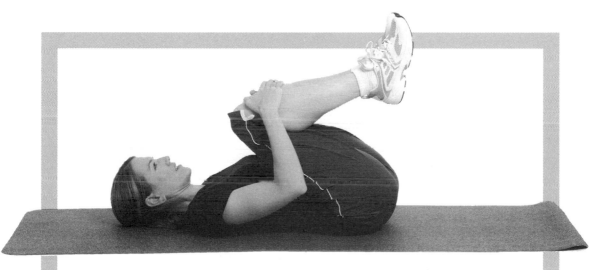

8. KNEES TO CHEST STRETCH
See directions on page 38 for this exercise, which is pictured above.

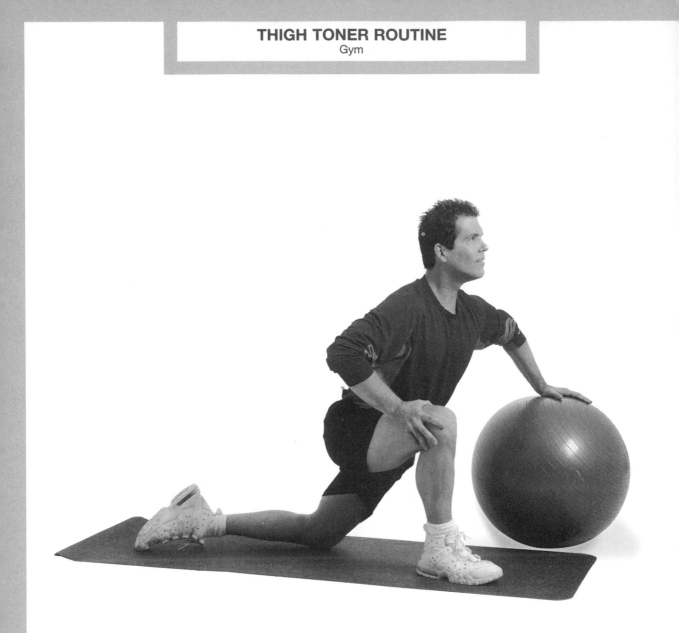

9. BALL HIP FLEXOR STRETCH
See directions on page 43 for this exercise, which is pictured above.

172

Summary for
Thigh Toner Routine: Gym

Exercise*	Workout Targets
Basic Squat Press	2–3 sets of 15 reps
Leg Press	2–3 sets of 8–15 reps
Hamstring Curls	2–3 sets of 8–15 reps
Stationary Dumbbell Lunge	2–3 sets of 8–15 reps (each side)
Heel Raises	2–3 sets of 15 reps
Straight-Leg Front Leg Lifts	2–3 sets of 8–15 reps (each side)
Floor "V" Center Stretch	2 times (hold for 10–15 seconds each time)
Knees to Chest Stretch	2 times (hold for 10–15 seconds each time)
Ball Hip Flexor Stretch	2 times (hold for 10–15 seconds each time on each side)

*Increase the resistance when the exercise begins to feel too easy.

WARM-UP

• 4–5 minutes on cardio equipment of choice, marching in place, or walking • 10 seconds of arm circles to the front; 10 seconds of arm circles to the back • 12 high knee lifts (alternate 6 per side)

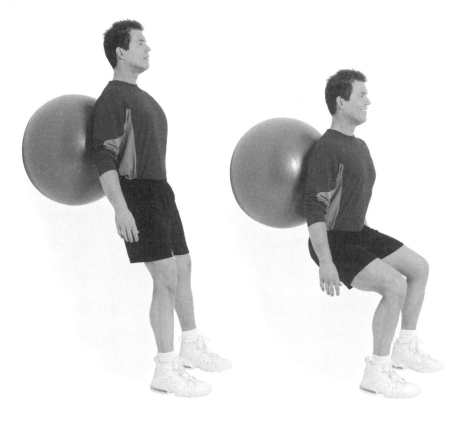

1. BALL WALL SQUAT PRESS

See directions on page 134 for this exercise, which is pictured above.

174

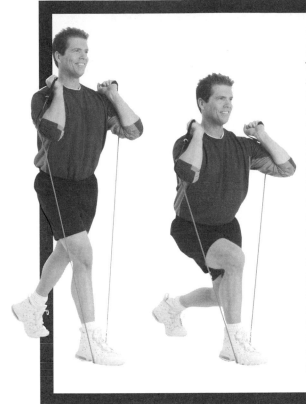

2. TUBING LUNGE
(PRESSING MOTION)

Target: quadriceps, hamstrings, glutes, and entire hip area

Positioning: Place one foot over the center of the tubing and the other foot 1–2 feet behind you in a split stance. Make sure your feet are firmly planted on the floor. The heel of your back foot will be slightly off the floor. Grasp the tubing handles in your hands. Keep your shoulders and back straight. Activate your supercenter. Keep your shoulders back and your face straight ahead.

Motion: In a controlled manner, bend your knees in a comfortable range of motion (not past 90 degrees) into a lunge position, keeping your front knee in line with your ankle (so as not to let your knee jut forward), as shown. Slowly return to the original position. Continue the exercise for the recommended number of repetitions. Repeat on the other leg.

3. BALL BRIDGE (PRESSING MOTION)

Target: hamstrings, glutes, quadriceps, hip adductors and abductors, deep core, and pelvic muscles

Positioning: Plant your feet firmly on the ground. Lie faceup with the ball placed in your mid- to upper back, shoulder, and neck area. This positioning gives your neck and shoulders full support and alleviates unnecessary stress. Your neck should be in a neutral position, keeping your head from dropping backward or your chin from dropping down. Align your hips, knees, and ankles for maximum stability.

Motion: Lower your hips straight down to the floor in a controlled manner. Then raise them toward the ceiling until your upper legs are parallel to the floor. Keep your knees directly over your ankles so your legs do not move inward or outward. This helps keep the ball absolutely stable. Continue for recommended number of repetitions.

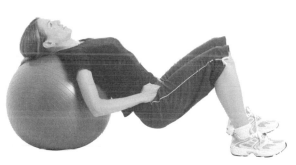

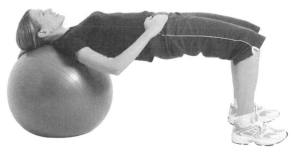

175

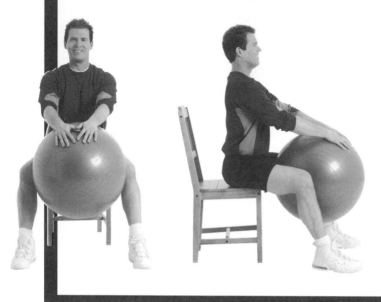

4. BALL SQUEEZE
(PRESSING MOTION)
Target: inner thigh muscles

Positioning: Sit up nice and tall with your feet firmly planted on the floor. Place the ball between your legs, as shown.

Motion: Press your legs toward each other, squeezing the ball. Return to the original position and repeat for desired reps. You determine the amount of resistance for this exercise by how hard you squeeze the ball.

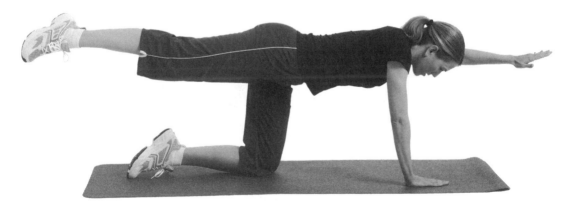

5. QUADRIPED (CORE)
Target: hip area, core, and shoulders

Positioning: Begin on your hands and knees, then take the position shown above. Fully extend one arm and the opposite leg. Activate your supercenter while keeping your back straight and facing down for optimum neck alignment.

Motion: Hold this position for 10–20 seconds, then repeat on the opposite side.

6. HEEL RAISES (PRESSING MOTION)
See directions on page 169 for this exercise.

7. STRAIGHT-LEG FRONT LEG LIFTS
See directions on page 170 for this exercise.

8. FLOOR "V" CENTER STRETCH
See directions on page 44 for this exercise.

9. KNEES TO CHEST STRETCH
See directions on page 38 for this exercise.

10. BALL HIP FLEXOR STRETCH
See directions on page 43 for this exercise.

Summary for
Thigh Toner Routine: Home

Exercise*	Workout Targets
Ball Wall Squat Press	2–3 sets of 8–15 reps
Tubing Lunge	2–3 sets of 8–15 reps (each side)
Ball Bridge	2–3 sets 8–15 reps
Ball Squeeze	2–3 sets 8–15 reps
Quadriped	2–3 sets of 15 reps (each side)
Heel Raises	2–3 sets 8–15 reps
Straight-Leg Front Leg Lifts	2–3 sets 8–15 reps (each side)
Floor "V" Center Stretch	2 times (hold for 10–15 seconds each time)
Knees to Chest Stretch	2 times (hold for 10–15 seconds each time)
Ball Hip Flexor Stretch	2 times (hold for 10–15 seconds each time, each side)

*Increase the resistance when the exercise begins to feel too easy.

WARM-UP

• 4–5 minutes on cardio equipment of choice, marching in place, or walking • 10 seconds of arm circles to the front; 10 seconds of arm circles to the back • 12 high knee lifts (alternate 6 per side)

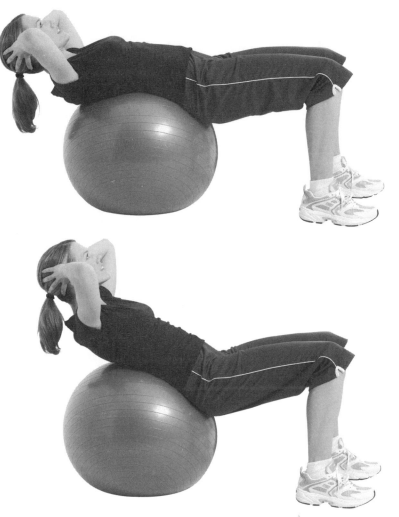

1. BALL CRUNCH (CORE)

Target: the entire abdominal region and comprehensive core

Positioning: Lie faceup on the stability ball with the ball placed at the mid- to low back. Plant your feet firmly on the floor and place your hands behind your head. Make sure your lower body is parallel to the floor.

Motion: Bring your chest toward your knees. Keep your hips and lower body stable. Slowly return to the original position and continue for the recommended number of repetitions.

178

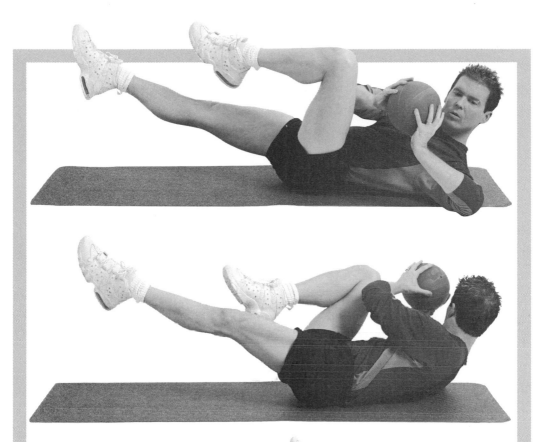

Tip: You can do this exercise without the medicine ball by placing your hands behind your head and bringing each elbow toward the opposite knee, as shown at right.

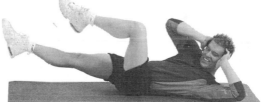

2. MEDICINE BALL FLOOR BICYCLES
(CORE AND ROTATING MOTION)

Target: the entire abdominal region and hip flexor areas

Positioning: Lie faceup on floor with your knees slightly bent. Hold the medicine ball in both hands above your chest.

Motion: Bring your left knee toward your chest while simultaneously rotating the right side of your upper body and the ball toward your left knee. At the same time, fully extend your right leg. Continue this motion, alternating sides for the recommended number of repetitions. (Each time you extend your leg It counts as one repetition.) Concentrate on keeping the motion fluid.

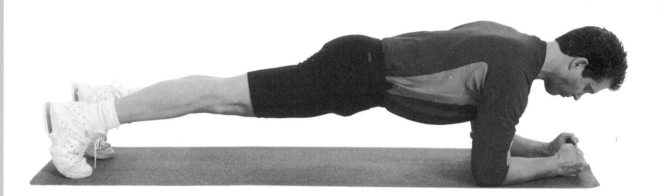

3. PLANKS (CORE)

Target: Comprehensive core, shoulders

Positioning: Assume the position shown above with your weight supported on your toes, elbows, and forearms. Make sure your elbows are directly under your shoulders. Your feet should be slightly apart. Keep your head in alignment with your spine.

Motion: Hold this position for 10–20 seconds while breathing normally.

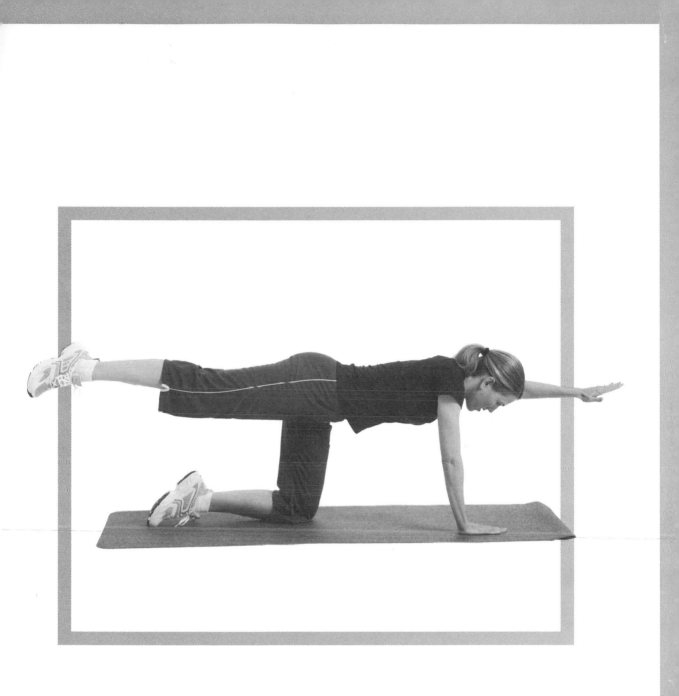

4. QUADRIPED (CORE)
See directions on page 176 for this exercise, which is pictured above.

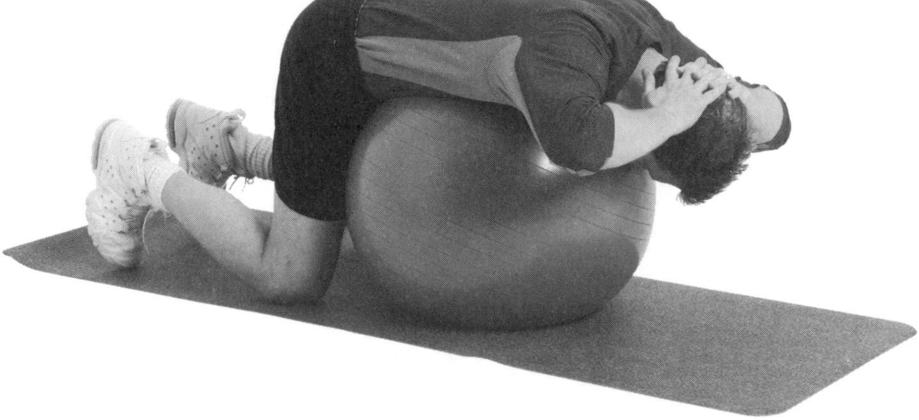

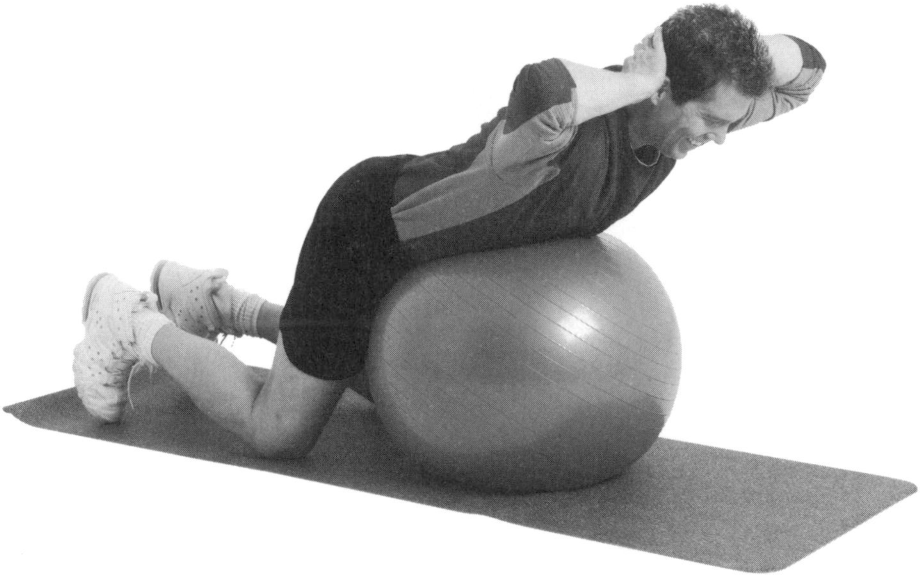

5. REVERSE BALL CRUNCH (CORE)

Target: low back, upper back, and spinal erectors

Positioning: Place your body over the stability ball, facedown, with hands behind your head, as shown.

Motion: Raise your upper body to a comfortable but challenging level but no higher than shown above. You will feel this in the low back area; it is the opposite motion of an abdominal crunch. Lower slowly to the original position and continue for the recommended number of repetitions.

182

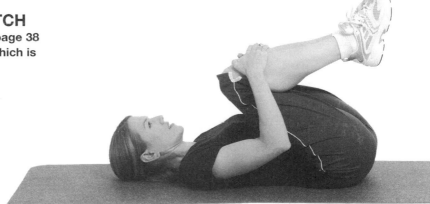

6. WASHING MACHINES (CORE AND ROTATING MOTION)

Target: core and shoulders

Positioning: Plant your feet firmly on the floor. Hold the medicine ball (or dumbbell) out in front of you. Activate your supercenter.

Motion: Rotate to your right side. Outstretch both arms, holding the medicine ball high up toward your right side. Swing the ball down and around, then go high up and over to the opposite side. Continue on both sides for the recommended number of repetitions.

7. KNEES TO CHEST STRETCH

See directions on page 38 for this exercise, which is pictured at right.

183

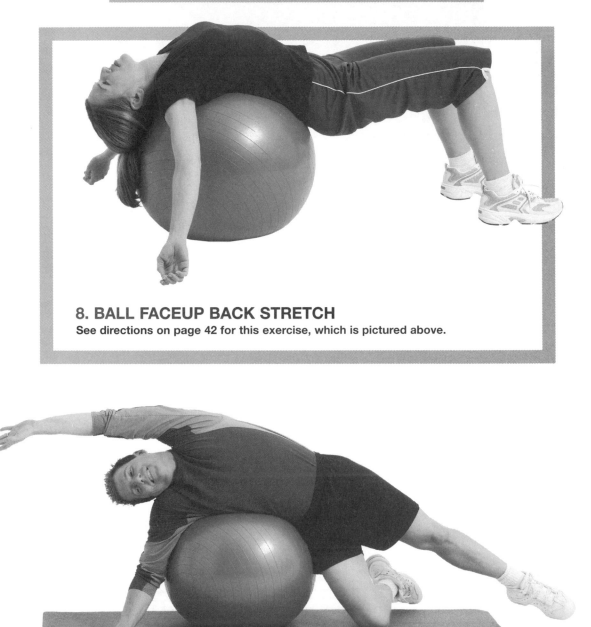

8. BALL FACEUP BACK STRETCH
See directions on page 42 for this exercise, which is pictured above.

9. SIDE-LYING BALL STRETCH
See directions on page 41 for this exercise, which is pictured above.

Summary for
Ab Tightening Core Routine

Exercise*	Workout Targets
Ball Crunch	2–3 sets of 15 reps
Mcdicine Ball Floor Bicycles	2–3 sets of 20 reps (each extension of the leg is one rep)
Planks	2–3 times (hold 10–20 seconds)
Quadriped	2 times (hold 20 seconds, each side)
Reverse Ball Crunch	2–3 sets of 8–12 reps
Washing Machines	2–3 sets of 12 (6 to each side)
Knees to Chest Stretch	2 times (hold 10–15 seconds)
Ball Faceup Back Stretch	2 times (hold 10–15 seconds)
Side-Lying Ball Stretch	2 times (hold 10–15 seconds, each side)

*Increase the resistance when the exercise begins to feel too easy.

WARM-UP

• 4–5 minutes on cardio equipment of choice, marching in place, or walking • 10 seconds of arm circles to the front; 10 seconds of arm circles to the back • 12 high knee lifts (alternate 6 per side)

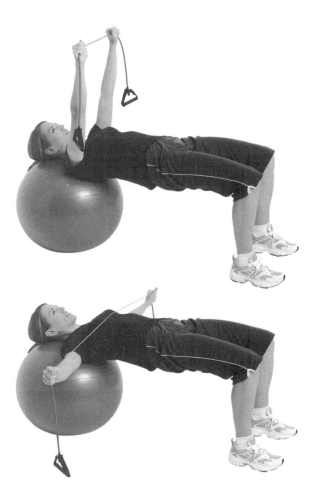

1. BALL TUBING PULL-APARTS (PULLING MOTION)

Target: chest and pecs

Positioning: Lie faceup on the stability ball with your head, neck, and shoulders rested on the ball and your upper legs parallel to the floor. Holding the tubing in each hand, raise your arms straight above you, perpendicular to the floor.

Motion: Open your arms to the sides until they are even with your torso. Keep your arms rigid and straight throughout the motion, but do not lock your elbows. Return your arms to the original position and continue for the recommended number of repetitions.

186

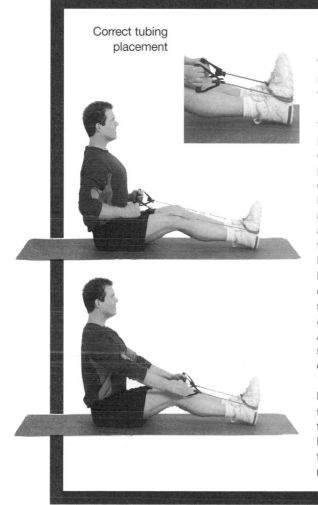

Correct tubing placement

2. SEATED TUBING ROW
(PULLING MOTION)

Target: lats, rhomboids, mid trapezius, rear deltoids, and biceps (muscles of the back and elbow flexors)

Positioning: Sit on the floor and wrap the tubing around both feet so it is placed in the middle of each foot and coming up the outside of your legs. Then pass the tubing again across the middle of the feet, coming up the outside of the legs to secure the tubing. (See the photo, above left, for correct placement.) Grasp a handle in each hand and make sure that both sides of the tubing are equal in length to provide the same resistance on both sides. Sit up nice and tall with your arms fully extended. Keep your knees slightly bent throughout the exercise. For added comfort use a cushion or pillow. Activate your supercenter for back support. You can sit against the wall for even more back support.

Motion: Bring your elbows back directly beside your body to just past your shoulders. Squeeze your shoulder blades together at the end of the motion. Release, fully extending your arms back to the original position. Continue for the recommended number of repetitions.

3. STANDING TUBING CHEST PUSH
See the directions on page 102 for this exercise.

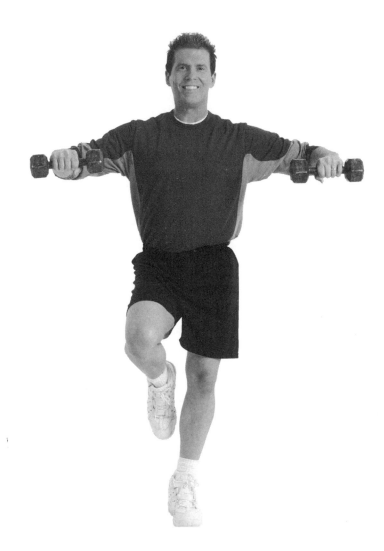

4. STANDING DUMBBELL LATERAL RAISE (SINGLE-LEG OPTION)
See the directions on page 126 for this exercise, which is pictured above.

Summary for
Upper-Body Balance Routine

Exercise*	Workout Targets
Ball Tubing Pull-Aparts	2–3 sets of 15 reps
Seated Tubing Row	2–3 sets of 15 reps
Standing Tubing Chest Push	2–3 sets of 15 reps
Standing Dumbbell Lateral Raise (Single-Leg Option)	2–3 sets of 15 reps

*Increase the resistance when the exercise begins to feel too easy.

WARM-UP

• 4–5 minutes on cardio equipment of choice, marching in place, or walking • 10 seconds of arm circles to the front; 10 seconds of arm circles to the back • 12 high knee lifts (alternate 6 per side)

1. FLAT BENCH DUMBBELL CHEST PUSH

See the directions on page 142 for this exercise.

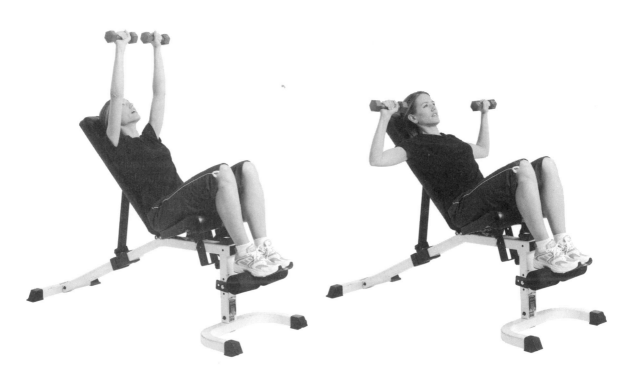

2. INCLINE DUMBBELL CHEST PUSH

Target: upper chest, shoulders, and triceps

Positioning: Lie faceup on the bench with your head rested on the upholstery. Hold a dumbbell in each hand. Fully extend your arms toward the ceiling, perpendicular to the floor. Your feet may rest on the equipment's pads, as shown, or flat on the floor if the bench is low enough to the ground.

Motion: Bend your elbows to approximately a 90-degree angle with your elbows dipping slightly lower than your shoulders. Extend your elbows back to the beginning position by pushing the dumbbells straight up toward the ceiling. Continue for the recommended number of repetitions.

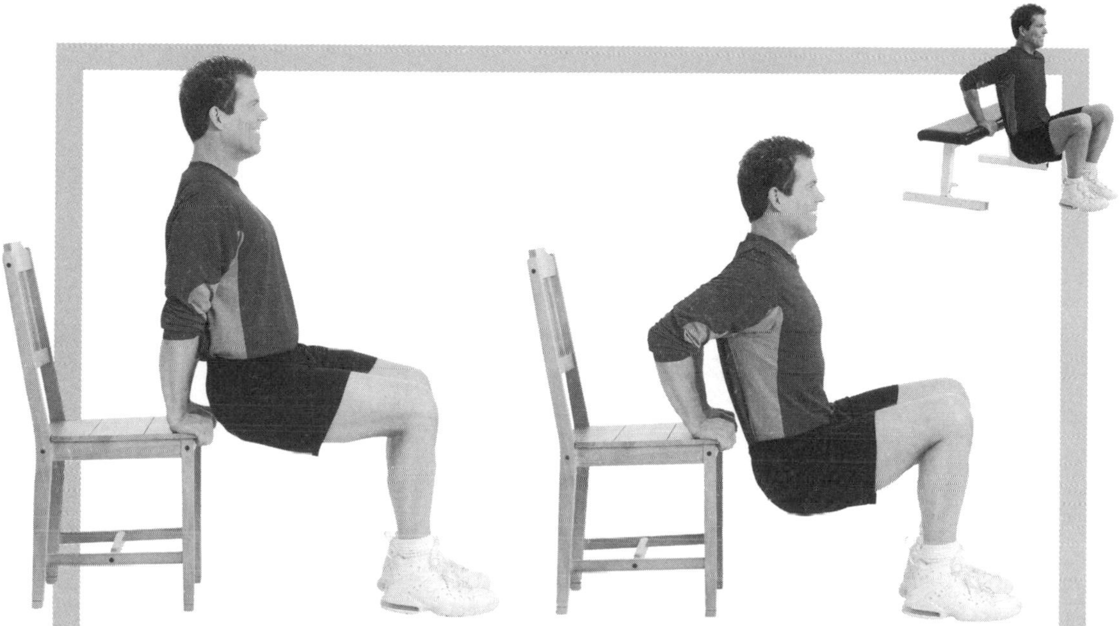

3. BENCH OR CHAIR DIPS (PUSHING MOTION)

Target: shoulders and triceps

Positioning: Stand with your feet flat on the floor and your knees bent at a 90-degree angle. Place your hands securely on the chair or bench with your arms fully extended, as shown above left. Keep your shoulders back and down. Look straight ahead, not down.

Motion: Bend your elbows to a maximum of a 90-degree angle as you lower your body toward the floor. Press up to the original position and continue for the recommended number of repetitions. Do not let your elbows lock.

4. STANDING OVERHEAD DUMBBELL PUSH

See the directions on page 125 for this exercise.

5. STANDING DUMBBELL LATERAL RAISE (PUSHING MOTION)

See the directions on page 126 for this exercise.

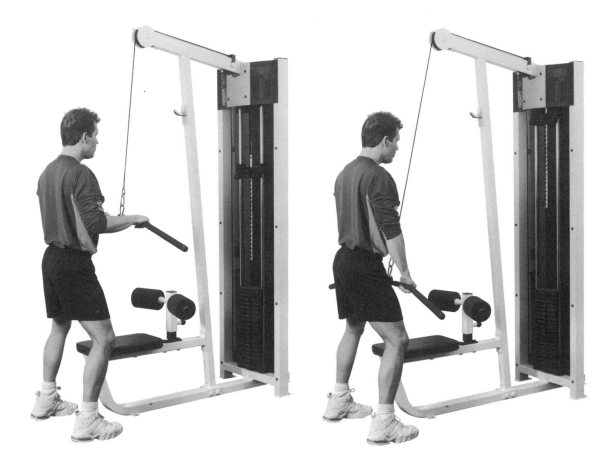

6. TRICEPS PRESS-DOWN (PUSHING MOTION)

Target: triceps

Positioning: Stand directly below the high pulley, as shown. Plant your feet firmly on the floor and bend your knees. Activate your supercenter. Place your elbows directly beside you at a 90-degree angle. Keep your wrists straight.

Motion: Extend your lower arm down to a straightened position. Return to the beginning position. Continue for the recommended number of repetitions.

Tip: Try this exercise while standing on one leg to incorporate balance and core work.

192

Summary for Upper-Body Focus Routine #1: Pushing/Gym

Exercise*	Workout Targets
Flat Bench Dumbbell Chest Push	2–3 sets of 8–15 reps
Incline Dumbbell Chest Push	2–3 sets of 8–15 reps
Bench or Chair Dips	2–3 sets of 8–15 reps
Standing Overhead Dumbbell Push	2–3 sets of 8–15 reps
Standing Dumbbell Lateral Raise	2–3 sets of 8–15 reps
Triceps Press-Down	2–3 sets of 8–15 reps

*Increase the resistance when the exercise begins to feel too easy.

WARM-UP

• 4–5 minutes on cardio equipment of choice, marching in place, or walking • 10 seconds of arm circles to the front; 10 seconds of arm circles to the back • 12 high knee lifts (alternate 6 per side)

1. SEATED LAT PULLDOWN
See the directions on page 143 for this exercise.

2. SEATED ROW (PULLING MOTION)
See the directions on page 143 for this exercise.

3. BALL TUBING PULL-APARTS (PULLING MOTION)
See the directions on page 186 for this exercise.

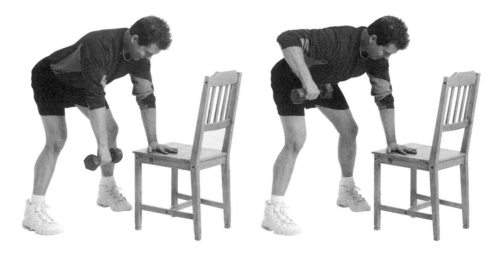

4. SINGLE-ARM DUMBBELL PULL (HIGH)
Target: upper and mid back, rear shoulder, biceps (elbow flexors), and core

Position: Begin with your knees slightly bent with one hand on a chair or bench for added stability. Grasp a dumbbell with the other hand (the working side) and extend this arm towards the floor. Keep your upper body almost parallel to the floor, as shown. Look down to assure optimum neck alignment. Draw your naval in toward your spine to activate your supercenter. Keep your body stable throughout the exercise.

Motion: Pull the dumbbell up in the plane of motion that is just below the shoulder. Your elbow will top out at approximately a 90-degree angle. Next, extend the dumbbell back down to the starting position. Continue the exercise for the recommended number of reps, then immediately repeat on the other side.

Tip: In the Single-Arm Dumbbell Pull (Low) on page 120, the elbow comes up directly beside the body. Notice how in this Single-Arm Dumbbell Pull (High), the elbow is coming up more toward the plane of motion of the shoulder.

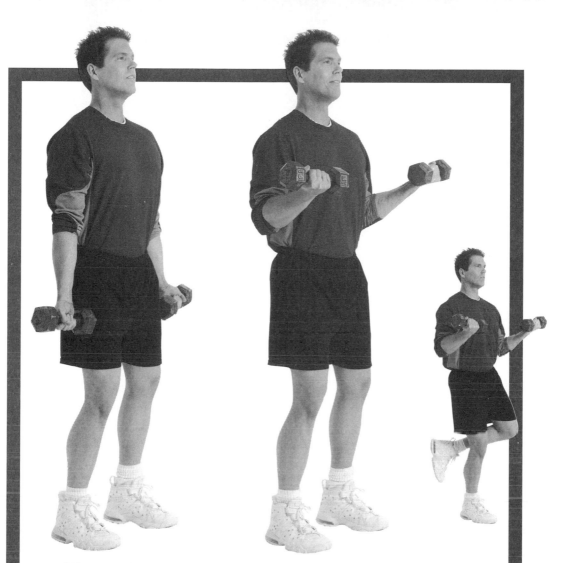

5. STANDING DUMBBELL ARM CURLS (PULLING MOTION)

Target: biceps, elbow flexors, core

Positioning: Stand nice and tall with your feet firmly planted on the floor and your knees bent. Grasp a dumbbell in each hand and let your arms hang naturally to your side with palms facing front. Activate your supercenter.

Motion: Bend your lower arms until your elbow goes just beyond a 90-degree angle. Slowly return to the original position. Continue for the recommended number of repetitions. Make sure to keep your shoulders, torso, and elbows absolutely stable throughout the exercise so as not to let your body waver.

Tip: You may perform this exercise on one leg, as shown far right, for added core and balance work.

Summary for Upper-Body Focus Routine #1: Pulling/Gym

Exercise*	Workout Targets
Seated Lat Pulldown	2–3 sets of 8–15 reps
Seated Row	2–3 sets of 8–15 reps
Ball Tubing Pull-Aparts	2–3 sets of 8–15 reps
Single-Arm Dumbbell Pull (High)	2–3 sets of 8–15 reps (each side)
Standing Dumbbell Arm Curls	2–3 sets of 8–15 reps

*Increase the resistance when the exercise begins to feel too easy.

Perform each of the following stretches twice after both the Upper Body Focus Routine #1 and Upper Body Focus Routine #2.

STANDING PEC/SHOULDER STRETCH
See the directions on page 150 for this exercise.

STANDING SHOULDER STRETCH
See the directions on page 35 for this exercise.

STANDING LAT STRETCH
See the directions on page 151 for this exercise.

NECK STRETCH
See the directions on page 36 for this exercise.

WARM-UP

• 4–5 minutes on cardio equipment of choice, marching in place, or walking • 10 seconds of arm circles to the front; 10 seconds of arm circles to the back • 12 high knee lifts (alternate 6 per side)

1. KNEE OR STANDARD PUSH-UP
See the directions on page 119 for this exercise.

2. BALL CHEST PUSH
See the directions on page 132 for this exercise.

3. STANDING TUBING OVERHEAD PUSH
See the directions on page 113 for this exercise.

4. STANDING TUBING LATERAL RAISE (PUSHING MOTION)
See the directions on page 114 for this exercise.

5. BENCH OR CHAIR DIPS (PUSHING MOTION)
See the directions on page 191 for this exercise.

Summary for Upper-Body Focus Routine #2: Pushing/Home

Exercise*	Workout Targets
Knee or Standard Push-Up	2–3 sets of 8–15 reps
Ball Chest Push	2–3 sets of 8–15 reps
Standing Tubing Overhead Push	2–3 sets of 8–15 reps
Standing Tubing Lateral Raise	2–3 sets of 8–15 reps
Bench or Chair Dips	2–3 sets of 8–15 reps

*Increase the resistance when the exercise begins to feel too easy.

WARM-UP

• 4–5 minutes on cardio equipment of choice, marching in place, or walking • 10 seconds of arm circles to the front; 10 seconds of arm circles to the back • 12 high knee lifts (alternate 6 per side)

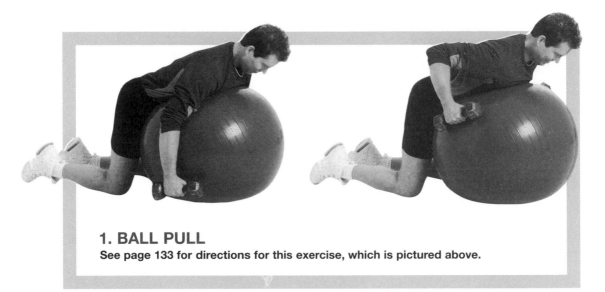

1. BALL PULL
See page 133 for directions for this exercise, which is pictured above.

2. SEATED TUBING ROW (PULLING MOTION)
See the directions on page 187 for this exercise.

3. STANDING TUBING PULL-APARTS (PULLING MOTION)

Target: chest and pecs

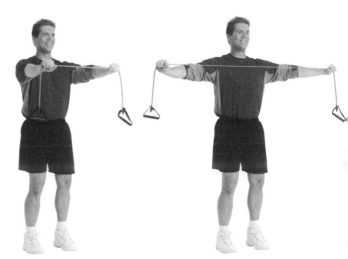

Position: Stand nice and tall with feet firmly planted on the ground and knees slightly bent. Place the tubing in both hands and reach your arms out directly in front of you as shown. Your elbows remain fully extended at chest level (do not bend them), but do not "lock" the elbows.

Motion: Simply move your arms out to the side as the tubing stretches directly in front of your chest, as shown. Return the arms to the opening position and repeat for desired reps.

Tip: **To increase the level of difficulty and incorporate core and balance work, stand on a single leg while doing this exercise.**

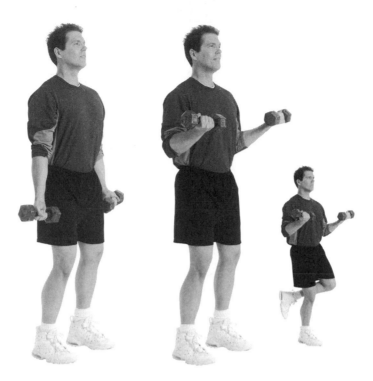

4. STANDING DUMBBELL ARM CURLS (PULLING MOTION)
See the directions on page 195 for this exercise, which is pictured above.

Summary for Upper-Body Focus Routine #2: Pulling/Home

Exercise*	Workout Targets
Ball Pull	2–3 sets of 8–15 reps
Seated Tubing Row	2–3 sets of 8–15 reps
Standing Tubing Pull-Aparts	2–3 sets of 8–15 reps
Standing Dumbbell Arm Curls	2–3 sets of 8–15 reps

*Increase the resistance when the exercise begins to feel too easy.

WARM-UP

• 4–5 minutes on cardio equipment of choice, marching in place, or walking • 10 seconds of arm circles to the front; 10 seconds of arm circles to the back • 12 high knee lifts (alternate 6 per side)

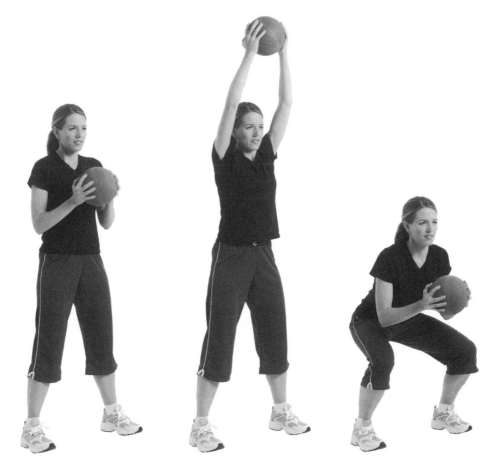

1. MEDICINE BALL SQUATS (PRESSING MOTION)

Target: lower body, core, and upper body.

Positioning: Stand nice and tall with your chest high and face forward. Plant your feet firmly on the floor with your feet slightly more than shoulder width apart. Activate your supercenter. Hold the medicine ball directly in front of you, as shown.

Motion: With both hands on the ball, reach up over your head (do not hyperextend your knee joint) with your arms fully extended, as shown. Then bend your knees to no more than 90 degrees into the squat position as you bring the ball back down to your midsection. The motion should be smooth, and you should not exceed a range that is not comfortable for you. Return to the original position. Continue for the recommended number of repetitions. For increased intensity, bring the ball down closer to the floor during the squat motion.

2. MEDICINE BALL SIDE LUNGES (PRESSING, CORE, AND ROTATING MOTION)

Target: hip area, hamstrings, quadriceps, and inner thighs

Positioning: Place your feet wider than shoulder width apart and bend your knees slightly. Hold the medicine ball in your hands. Keep your shoulders back—in other words, don't hunch over—and activate your supercenter.

Motion: Lunge sideways to your right, slightly rotating your upper body. Repeat this motion to your left. Continue this side-to-side motion for the recommended number of repetitions.

3. MEDICINE BALL FLOOR BICYCLES (CORE AND ROTATING MOTION)

See the directions on page 179 for this exercise.

4. WASHING MACHINES (CORE AND ROTATING MOTION)

See the directions on page 183 for this exercise.

5. KNEES TO CHEST STRETCH

See the directions on page 38 for this exercise.

6. BALL FACEUP BACK STRETCH

See the directions on page 42 for this exercise.

7. SIDE-LYING BALL STRETCH

See the directions on page 41 for this exercise.

Summary for Medicine Ball Routine

Exercise*	Workout Targets
Medicine Ball Squats	2–3 sets of 8–15 reps
Medicine Ball Side Lunges	2–3 sets of 8–16 reps (4–8 on each side)
Medicine Ball Floor Bicycles	2–3 sets of 20–30 reps (each leg extension is one rep)
Washing Machines	2–3 sets of 8–16 reps (4–8 on each side)
Knees to Chest Stretch	2 times (hold 10–15 seconds)
Ball Faceup Back Stretch	2 times (hold 10–15 seconds)
Side-Lying Ball Stretch	2 times (hold 10–15 seconds on each side)

*Increase the resistance when the exercise begins to feel too easy.

Beyond the First Eight Weeks:
More Metabolic Burst Training Options

If there's one thing I want you to remember about Metabolic Burst Training, it's this: Working out at *higher* intensity for *shorter* amounts of time gives you superior overall metabolic benefits versus working out at moderate intensity for one longer period. So if you'd like to incorporate more cardio work into your program, you should try to break up an hour-long workout into shorter segments that you tackle throughout your day. Breaking up your workouts into smaller chunks makes sense: Studies show that doing two 20- to 30-minute workouts in a day enables you to work at a higher intensity for each workout than you'd use in one 40- or 60-minute workout, resulting in far better calorie burning, fat burning, and overall metabolic benefit.

For optimum results from both your resistance and Metabolic Burst Training, refer to the guidelines on page 152. Burst Training is best performed immediately *after* your resistance training, on days you aren't doing resistance training, or in the afternoon or evening of a day when you do resistance training. If you do Burst Training in the morning, wait five or six hours before doing resistance work for optimum metabolic response.

The following exercise options can be done in place of the Metabolic Burst Training routine you used in the first eight weeks. It's a great way to "change it up" and keep your excitement about exercising high. Keep in mind that intensity is key. Work at *your individual* highest level on a given day. This level will change from day to day.

- **A 20–30 minute split routine** twice per day to total 40–60 minutes. I highly recommend this approach if you desire an intense day of cardio work.
- **A 30-minute all-out Metabolic Burst Training session.** It comprises the following: four- or five-minute warm-up, 20 minutes of full-intensity cardio (no intervals), and a five-minute cooldown and stretch.
- **A 20-minute all-out Burst Training session.** It comprises a four- to five-minute warm-up, 10 minutes of full-intensity cardio (no intervals), and five minutes of cooldown and stretch.
- **A 20- to 30-minute interval training sequence.** It comprises a four- to five-minute warm-up; 10- to 20-minutes of interval training, alternating 30-second "sprints" with 30-second "cruises"; and a 5-minute cooldown and stretch.
- **An all-out five- or 10-minute burst of cardio** done *after* any one of the resistance training routines in Chapter 6 or the spot-conditioning routines in this chapter. You are already warmed up, so just go for it!

- **Finally, incorporate the shorter workout segments described** in "Beyond the First Four Weeks" (see page 156). Remember that 30 minutes of work split into smaller increments throughout the day (three 10-minute or two 15-minute workouts) will produce the *same or better* results than 30 minutes of work done in one chunk. That's because you get that metabolic blast at several points throughout your day.
- **Be creative!** Use your imagination to come up with different combinations that suit your time frame, venue, or individual level on that day. The sky is the limit here!

Family Activities for Lifetime Fitness

I want to talk about something that will truly enhance the quality of your life and relationships: having fun with fitness as a family. If you're a parent like I am, you must pay close attention to the health and fitness of your children and set a good example. It is vital that we teach and encourage our kids to stay active, because active kids become active adults—plain and simple. It's no secret that overeating and lack of physical activity can lead to a host of potentially life-threatening problems. Present couch potatoes make future couch potatoes.

Exercising with your kids is a fantastic opportunity for parents. It establishes a great sense of camaraderie and companionship, and it's a time to bond with your children. This is time well spent. My wife used to jog with her dad when she was younger. She learned good habits from her father, and she now maintains a healthy lifestyle. And her dad is now 82 years old and still exercising three times per week! When I was a child, my father made me a weight bench out of wood. We lifted weights together twice a week. This inspired me to always include exercise in my life. As parents we set the example by presenting a positive image of health, fitness, and wellness. And you not only send your children this positive message, but you stay fit yourself!

Try setting aside two hours per week to exercise with your children. You can do it early in the morning (before school and work), in the evening just before dinner, or on weekends. I suggest that you "schedule" these activities to ensure that nothing interferes with your workout plans. Find activities that you both really enjoy so you'll look forward to doing them on a regular basis.

Some examples may include:

- Weight lifting or cardio work in your home gym or at the health club, recreation center, or YMCA

- Biking
- Hiking
- Playing catch or hitting fly balls or grounders at the park
- Shooting baskets or practicing another team sport, such as soccer or volleyball
- Taking a walk or jog outside
- Going to the track and practicing track events
- Heavy bag work or martial arts
- Tai Chi or yoga
- Golf (walk the course)
- Tennis
- Swimming
- Aerobics classes or tapes
- Father-son or mother-daughter church, recreation, or sport leagues

You may have slightly different preferences, in which case you could combine any of these or other activities together. For example, Dad is in the garage lifting weights while son or daughter is on the treadmill, riding a stationary bike, or shooting hoops in the driveway. Or Mom and Dad are doing yoga while son or daughter is practicing on the heavy bag or running wind sprints. Then you both go out for a walk or bike ride to complete the workout.

The point is that you have set times to work out together. There is so much value in this time together. Follow these workouts with a healthy meal or snack and talk to your kids about healthy nutrition and devoting time for exercise. For most kids a key time for exercise and physical activity is after school. Even with a boatload of homework, 30 minutes to an hour of some form of exercise will only enhance study time. Consistently parking in front of the TV or diving into the latest video game after school with a tub of ice cream would not be my recommendation, nor is it a good prestudy regimen!

Many kids lose interest in sports or physical activity if they don't make the team or are consistently chosen last for playground events. Schools and the media tend to put a huge emphasis on external motivation and competition instead of focusing on the pure joy of exercise and sport, along with the health and wellness benefits of leading an active lifestyle. Only a select few make the team. What about everybody else? I always say that more emphasis needs to be placed on "personal bests" and continued individual improvement. Be in competition with yourself. Sometimes children get discouraged if they don't live up to *your* standards as well. So again make sure activities are done in the name of fun, health, fitness, and wellness—not some test or standard you have set. Put the focus simply on giving the best that you can on a given day.

If you think about it, adults aren't spending hours in the gym each week because they want to be the best treadmill walker or weight lifter in the facility. We don't join the summer softball league because we think we're Barry Bonds or ride a bike because we're thinking of entering the Tour de France. We do these things to get a good workout, to be healthy, and to improve our quality of life. This is the mind-set we need to teach our kids early on. Don't wait until there is a weight problem. An active lifestyle needs to be a way of life. It is a mind-set, and it's up to us as parents to establish this from the get-go.

If you don't have children, encourage a friend, significant other, or spouse to be an exercise partner and join you in your weight loss efforts. But your partner must be absolutely committed to success. Sharing your journey to optimal health, fitness, and weight loss success can help you reach your goals. Still, on any given day, regardless of your partner's commitment or mood, you must stay totally focused and in the game.

If you'd like to be an active adult—or step up your activity level—this is the perfect time and opportunity to get it going and get moving. Not tomorrow, not next month, not when the weather gets better—the time is now.

> **"** Robert's "to-the-point" programs have continuously enabled me to increase my fitness level year after year. He is the consummate pro, always focused on my individual needs and goals. If I need a specific program or group of exercises to focus on my golf conditioning, Robert is there to plan and execute them. **"**
>
> **Jay Roth**
> NATIONAL EXECUTIVE DIRECTOR, DIRECTOR'S GUILD OF AMERICA

On-the-Road Travel Routine

There's no need to leave your workouts behind when you're traveling on business or vacation! The terrific benefit of tubing is that it is packable and fits well in a suitcase or briefcase. Take your copy of *Make Over Your Metabolism* with you. Here is a great *total body* travel workout to keep you in shape:

Standing Tubing Chest Push (page 102)	2-3 sets of 8–15 reps
Knee or Standard Push-Ups (page 119)	2-3 sets of 8–15 reps
Standing Tubing Lateral Raise (page 114)	2-3 sets of 8–15 reps
Single-Arm Tubing Pull (page 103)	2–3 sets of 8–15 reps each side
Seated Tubing Row (page 187)	2–3 sets of 8–15 reps
Tubing Squat Press (page 104)	2–3 sets of 8–15 reps
Tubing Lunge (page 175)	2–3 sets of 8–15 reps each side
Chair Bridge (page 105)	2–3 sets of 8–15 reps
Floor Bicycles without Medicine Ball (page 179)	2–3 sets of 24 reps
Superman (page 106)	2–3 times (hold for 10–15 seconds each)

Follow the above travel routine with the following stretches, performed twice:

Knees to Chest Stretch (page 38)
Seated Hamstring Stretch (page 37)
Standing Pec/Shoulder Stretch (page 150)
Standing Lat Stretch (page 151)

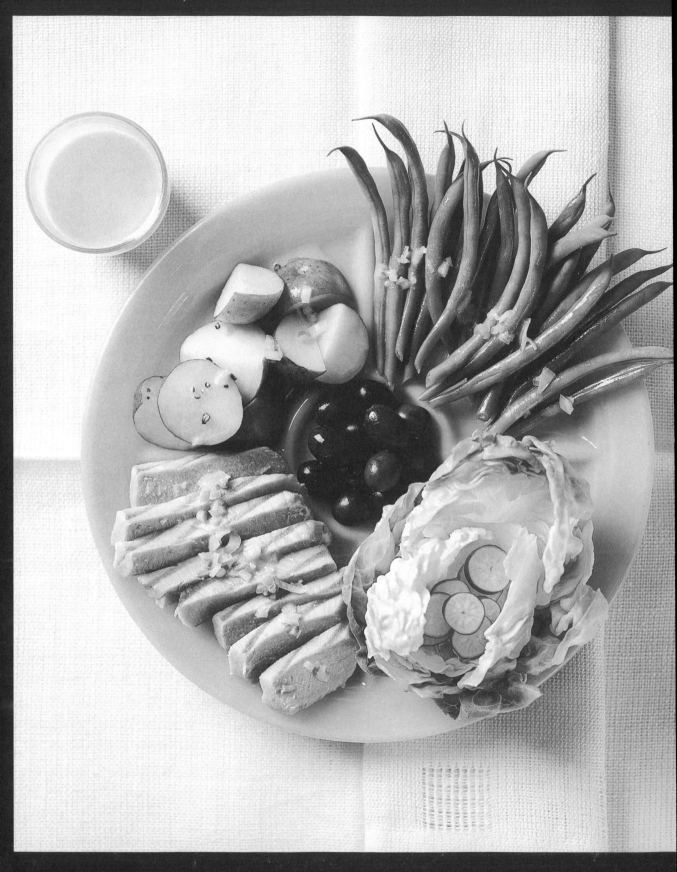

Chapter Eight

EXERCISING TO GIVE YOUR BODY AN AUTOMATIC METABOLIC BOOST IS ONLY ONE PART OF THE FAT-LOSS EQUATION. ANOTHER PART IS NUTRITION. YOU MUST TAKE CARE OF YOUR NUTRITIONAL NEEDS IN ORDER TO LOSE FAT AND get fit. And that doesn't mean just cutting back on junk food or going on some crazy crash diet. You need a plan of attack that's specifically designed to optimize your metabolism so you can get lean and stay that way.

In this chapter I'm going to lay down some key strategies that can definitely help you reach your goals. My Nutritional Life Plan is a simple approach that naturally boosts your metabolism, burns stored body fat, and helps you stay in optimum shape. On this eating plan you'll feel better and become healthier.

I know the first question on your mind is "What do I get to eat?" Turn the page to see a list of sanctioned foods and serving amounts I recommend on my Nutritional Life Plan. Get ready to learn how to build these foods into healthy meals and snacks.

The Nutritional Life Plan

The Nutritional Life Plan: Sanctioned Foods

Protein*

4 daily servings —at each meal and for 1 snack

Beef (ultra lean, 1–2 times per week max)	**Clams**	Grouper	**Red snapper**	Tuna
	Cod	**Haddock**	Salmon	**Turkey breast, ground**
Chicken breast, ground	**Cornish game hen**	Halibut	**Shark**	
		Lobster	Shrimp	Turkey breast, skin removed
Chicken breast, skin removed	Crab	Monkfish	**Sole**	
	Egg	**Orange roughy**	Tilapia	**Whey protein**
	Egg whites	Perch	**Tofu**	
	Flounder	**Pollock**	Trout	Whitefish
	Game meats			

Vegetables

Unlimited

Alfalfa sprouts	**Cabbage**	Eggplant	**Mustard greens**	Spinach
	Carrots	**Endive**	Okra	**Summer squash, all varieties**
Artichokes	**Cauliflower**	Garlic	**Onions**	
Arugula	Celery	**Green beans**	Parsley	Swiss chard
Asparagus	**Collard greens**	Green peas	**Pea pods**	**Tomatoes**
Beet greens	Cucumber	**Kale**	Peppers, all varieties	Turnip greens
Broccoli	**Dandelion greens**	Lettuce, all varieties	**Scallions**	**Watercress**
Brussels sprouts		**Mushrooms**		Zucchini

Starches

2 daily servings— breakfast and lunch mainly; no starches in the evening

Bagel (whole grain only)	**Bran muffin (high protein/high fiber only)**	Beans and legumes, including hummus and edamame (also high in protein)	**Millet**	Wild rice
Baked potato (with the skin)			Pumpkin	**Winter squash**
	Brown rice		**Quinoa**	
Baked sweet potato or yam	**Buckwheat**	**High-fiber cereals (such as Fiber One or All-Bran)**	Oatmeal, or virtually any whole grain hot cereal	Whole grain bread
	Corn			**Whole grain pasta (whole wheat, gluten-free, or spinach only)**
Barley	**Couscous**		**Wasa crackers**	

Fruits					
2 daily servings for the first 14 days; 3 daily servings thereafter	**Apple**	Boysenberries	Cranberries	Melon	**Plantain**
	Apricot	**Cantaloupe**	**Figs (fresh or dried)**	**Nectarines**	Plum
	Banana	Cherries		Papaya	**Pomegranate**
	Black currants	**Citrus fruits (oranges, grapefruit, tangerines, tangelos)**	Grapes	**Peaches**	Prunes
	Blackberries		**Guava**	Pear	**Raspberries**
	Blueberries		Kiwi fruit	**Persimmons**	Strawberries
			Mango	Pineapple	

Calcium-Rich Foods					
1–2 daily servings	**Almonds**	**Low-fat cottage cheese**	Fat-free or low-fat milk	**Feta cheese (low salt)**	**Fat-free, sugar-free yogurt**
	Low-fat cheeses			Goat cheese	

*Whenever possible, choose free-range, cage-free, hormone-free, and/or grass-fed protein sources.

Let's take a close look at each of these categories so you can learn to use food—which is the fuel that energizes you—to keep your metabolism up and running.

Protein

Delivering protein in precise doses throughout the day causes your body to burn an extra 150–200 calories a day. So you can look at eating protein as a way to burn calories! Why? Because protein stimulates the production of two appetite-regulating hormones, cholecystokinin and glucagon. Also, protein is made up of amino acids, which are harder for your body to break down, so you burn more calories processing them.

Protein is critical for controlling your appetite. If you ever find yourself feeling really hungry while trying to lose weight, this is a sign that your body is breaking down precious metabolism-boosting muscle. You certainly don't want that! To prevent it, you must put protein together with high-fiber foods such as vegetables and starches; this combination takes longer to digest, so you feel satisfied for a longer period of time. Protein plus fiber equals hunger control. Protein also helps balance your blood sugar, consequently taming cravings and keeping your body from losing muscle. Controlling cravings is a major component in maintaining permanent control over your weight. So you do really need to monitor your protein intake.

One protein serving looks like the size of a deck of cards.

Vegetables

The vegetables in the list on page 210 are actually a form of carbohydrate, the best source of energy for your body. Vegetables are packed with fiber, the indigestible part of plants that keeps your body processes regular. It's impossible to eat too many vegetables, especially because they are abundant sources of vitamins, minerals, antioxidants, and naturally occurring substances called phytochemicals, which are protective against a range of diseases.

Don't limit the size of your vegetable servings. You can fill up on these!

Starchy Carbohydrates

There are two kinds of carbohydrates: simple and complex. Starchy carbohydrates are a form of complex carbohydrates. You'll want to eat the complex kind, which includes starches, as well as vegetables and fruits. You'll want to avoid the simple kind, such as candy, cake, table sugar, syrups, soda, sweetened cereals, white bread, and white rice. Simple carbs are high in refined sugar and supply empty, non-nutritious calories. Even when modified to be low-carb, fat-free, or reduced-calorie, these foods are devoid of much nutrient value. Overeating simple carbs can result in excessive blood glucose increases, raise harmful triglyceride (blood fat) levels, and cause major weight gain, especially when eaten in excess. Keep them off of your shopping list and try to avoid these simple carbohydrate foods altogether.

You absolutely need natural, quality complex carbohydrates in your diet (these include the starches I've listed on page 210, as well as vegetables and fruits). They supply the primary source of fuel for your brain and muscles so they can operate properly.

Fiber Content of Key Foods

Food	Serving	Fiber (grams)
All-Bran (cereal)	1 ounce	8.5g
Almonds	**1 ounce**	**5g**
Apple	1 medium	3.2g
Banana	**1 medium**	**3g**
Blueberries	1 cup	3g
Bran muffin	**1**	**4g**
Broccoli	1 cup (cooked)	5g
Brown rice	**1 cup**	**3g**
Brussels sprouts	1 cup (cooked)	5g
Corn bran	**1 ounce**	**5.3g**
Edamame	½ cup (75g)	5g
Ezekiel bread	**1 slice (34g)**	**3g**
Figs	2	7.4g
Food For Life gluten-free bread	**1 slice (43g)**	**2g**
Green peas	1 cup (cooked)	5g
Lentil beans	**1 cup**	**9g**
Lima beans	1 cup (cooked)	7.5g
Muesli (cereal)	**½ cup**	**5g**
Orange	1 medium	2.8g
Pears	**1 medium**	**4g**
Pinto beans	1 cup (cooked)	9g
Raisins	**5 tablespoons**	**3g**
Raspberries	1 cup	9.2g
Spinach	**1 cup (cooked, 85g)**	**6.5g**
Sweet corn	1 cup (cooked)	4.7g
Wheat bran	**1 ounce**	**11.3g**
Whole green beans	¾ cup (85g)	2g
Whole wheat bagel	**1**	**2.7g**

Source: The Tufts University Guide to Nutrition

Starchy carbohydrates also help control your appetite, maintain steady blood sugar levels, and promote weight loss. They are rich in vital nutrients and fiber. Because fiber takes longer to digest, you feel full longer, particularly when you eat it with protein, as I've mentioned before. Think of this combination as a time-released energy source that prevents peaks and valleys in your blood sugar that can otherwise lead to food cravings. A great way to boost your fiber intake is to start the day with a cereal that has the word "bran" or "fiber" in the title.

I cannot stress enough the importance of fiber for overall health, blood sugar balance, and weight control. Americans do not consume enough fiber daily. I recommend a minimum of 25–50 grams daily, which depending on the source will be four to six servings per day. The chart on page 213 gives you a glimpse at some of the best fiber-rich foods. Include appropriate quantities of daily fiber in your food journal.

Another important word about carbohydrates: If you do not eat enough carbohydrates—which is what happens on low-carb diets—your body must draw energy from somewhere else, and the first place it turns to is your lean muscle. Because muscle dictates your metabolism, burning energy from it depletes that muscle and consequently puts the skids on your metabolism. So all those fat-burning fireplaces you've built through your resistance training start to go out, one by one. The investment you've made to burn optimum levels of fat 24-7, well, it starts bringing in a negative return. The message here: You need carbohydrates to drive your metabolism.

One starchy carbohydrate serving looks like one slice of bread; ½ cup of cereal, pasta, rice, pumpkin, or squash; one medium potato or sweet potato (about the size of a tennis ball).

Carbohydrates and Your Waistline

The type of carbohydrates you eat can affect the size of your belly. That's the latest word from scientists at Tufts University, who twice studied the effect of complex and simple carbs on waist circumference. In both studies individuals with the smallest increase in waist circumference ate mostly carbs rich in fiber, such as fruits, vegetables, and whole grains. On the other hand, those who ate a lot of refined carbs and processed foods had a much larger increase in their waist girth.

Waist size can be an indicator of abdominal fat, which has been linked to cardiovascular disease, premature death, stroke, type 2 (non-insulin dependent) diabetes, some cancers, and high blood pressure.

214

An expanding waistline also may be a symptom of metabolic syndrome, characterized by an aggregate of metabolic risk factors that include:

- Abdominal obesity (excessive fat tissue in and around the abdomen)
- Blood fat disorders such as high triglycerides, low HDL cholesterol, and high LDL cholesterol (all of which foster plaque buildup in artery walls)
- Elevated blood pressure
- Insulin resistance or glucose intolerance (which means that the body can't properly use insulin or blood sugar or insulin levels are elevated)
- A high level of inflammation in the body (as detected by elevated levels of C-reactive protein in the blood)

People with metabolic syndrome are at increased risk of coronary heart disease, stroke, and type 2 diabetes. This condition has become increasingly common in the United States, and it is estimated that more than 50 million Americans have it.

Fortunately metabolic syndrome can be prevented, even reversed, by changes in your lifestyle. These changes include losing body fat; following a low-fat, high-fiber diet; avoiding saturated and trans fats; eliminating or reducing sugars and processed foods; and increasing physical activity that includes resistance training and aerobic exercise. (Source: Egan, B.M. The Metabolic Syndrome. JANA, volume 8, 2005, pages 3–5.)

Fruits

Fresh fruits are among the most colorful and nutrient-packed foods you can eat. They're loaded with fiber (important for digestive health and reducing the risk of heart disease), and the flesh of fruits is rich in cancer-fighting antioxidants. Fruits also offer vitamin C, vitamin A, and potassium. They're just unbeatable when it comes to nutrition, plus as "nature's candy," they offer the best choice when you want something sweet.

I want to steer you away from fruit juices. My family used to own a house with two orange trees in the yard. So we'd make juice. It took as many as 12 oranges to squeeze a glass of juice. I thought to myself: I'd certainly rather eat one or two oranges than have to gulp down 10 or 12 of them in juice form. By eating whole fruits and avoiding juices, I guarantee you'll get fuller much faster. (That's because there is very little fiber in fruit juice.) You'll also take in much less sugar, so your blood sugar levels will stay much more stable.

One exception to this guideline is pomegranate juice. It is extremely high in antioxidants and has been shown in research to reduce blood pressure. I highly recommend that you enjoy this juice a few times a week as part of your fruit selection.

One fruit serving looks like one piece of fresh fruit or one cup of berries, grapes, or cherries.

Calcium-Rich Foods

Calcium continues to stay in the nutritional spotlight. New studies show it can be a weight-loss tool—not to mention that it is a crucial building block of healthy bones and teeth. It also has been shown to reduce the risk of high blood pressure, kidney stones, cardiovascular disease, and colon cancer.

Low-fat or nonfat milk, low-fat or nonfat cheese, and other dairy products are great sources of calcium. In fact the low-fat versions are up to 20 percent higher in calcium than whole-milk products.

If you're not a milk drinker, you can consume some calcium just by adding a few almonds to your snacks each day. Five to 10 almonds with a piece of fruit is a nice snack serving. Almonds contain other important nutrients as well, including vitamin E, magnesium, copper, and dietary fiber. A study conducted at the School of Public Health at Loma Linda University in California found that including some almonds in your diet can reduce your heart attack risk by as much as 50 percent. I *always* tote around a pack of organic almonds as my "emergency food."

One serving of calcium-rich foods looks like 1 cup of fat-free or low-fat milk or yogurt; ½ cup of low-fat cottage cheese; or a piece of cheese the size of a domino.

"Thin Fats" Versus "Fat Fats"

A diet that contains moderate levels of fat—as opposed to a strict low-fat diet—imay result in more long-term weight loss. Also important: Diets too low in fat tend to result in poor hormone production, which leads to a slower metabolism.

"Thin Fats" Choose these ...	"Fat Fats" ... and limit or avoid these
Canola oil	Bacon fat
Flaxseed oil	**Butter**
Ground flax meal	Cream, including half-and-half
Macadamia nut oil	**Lard**
Olive oil	Marbled fat in cuts of beef
Omega-3 fatty acids (found mostly in fish)	**Margarine**
Peanut, almond, and other natural nut butters	Shortening
Peanut oil	**Sour cream (use non-fat sour cream)**
Salad dressings, low-fat	
Sesame oil	
Trans-free fats and spreads	
Walnuts and walnut oil	

a slower metabolism.

Fats are another nutritional tool you can use to feel full longer and minimize blood sugar surges. The key is to choose healthier monounsaturated fats—the kind found in olive oil and canola oil—instead of saturated fats (found mostly in animal foods). Research suggests that monounsaturated fats burn a little faster than the saturated variety. Also include plenty of omega-3 fatty acids in your diet from sources such as cold-water fish (tuna, salmon, mackerel, and herring, among others).

To clarify which fats are best to include in your diet, I categorize fats into "thin fats" (those that are good for your metabolism and healthy for your body) and "fat fats" (those that tend to stick around in your body, make you fat, and cause disease). Clearly the consumption of the thin fats accelerates the loss of the fat fats. With this in mind here's a closer look at how to choose fats wisely.

Besides avoiding saturated fats, it's a good idea to steer clear of trans fats too. What is a trans fat? Without going into too much chemistry, a trans fat is a liquid unsaturated fat that has been transformed into a solid through a process called hydrogenation in order to stabilize the flavor of a product and give it a longer shelf life. Trans fats are baked goods, fried foods, and many processed foods.

Trans fats have been shown to raise levels of LDL (the "bad" artery-clogging form of cholesterol) and cause damage to cells. Eating trans fats is like throwing battery acid into your body. It's not healthy!

Fortunately the Food and Drug Administration (FDA) requires food manufacturers to list trans fats on the Nutrition Facts panel on their packaging. This move is designed to help us make healthier food choices, but it could also encourage food makers to reduce or abandon the use of trans fats, and that would be a good thing.

One "thin fat" serving looks like 1 to 2 tablespoons of oil or spreads.

How to Trim the Fat

Do you want some great ideas for reducing the fat content in foods without sacrificing taste or enjoyment? Try these suggestions:

- Broil, grill, or microwave meats, fish, and poultry, rather than fry them.
- Drain off the fat after you cook proteins.
- Baste your meat with wine or nonfat salad dressings instead of drippings.
- Trim all visible fat from meat and poultry before cooking.
- Use lemon juice to flavor steamed vegetables like broccoli or green beans.
- Instead of adding butter or oil, sprinkle cooked spinach with balsamic vinegar for extra zing and no added calories.
- Sprinkle steamed vegetables with fresh or dried herbs.
- Sauté vegetables in a little fat-free broth or lemon juice or lime juice.
- Use a nonstick pan so added fat won't be necessary, or use vegetable cooking spray on a regular pan.

Meals and Your Metabolism

Now that we've looked at exactly what you'll be eating, I want to talk about some key nutritional strategies that will accentuate your metabolism so you continue to burn optimum amounts of fat 24-7. When you fold these principles into your life, along with your resistance training and Metabolic Burst Training, you'll be on the road to getting the body you want. These strategies will fill you up while slimming you down.

Time Your Carbohydrates

Eating high-quality carbohydrates such as whole grains, fruits, and vegetables actually increases your metabolism, whereas slashing good carbs slows your metabolism down, according to research. Remember that the muscle on your body is fat-burning metabolic machinery. Without ample carbohydrates the first source your body will attack for its energy needs is your lean stores of precious muscle. So you don't want to go low-carb, but you do want to time your carbohydrate intake and choose only the healthiest carbs.

Your first meal of the day should contain your biggest carbohydrate intake. When you wake up, the stored carbs in your muscles (glycogen) are emptied; resupplying them is crucial for igniting your metabolic fireplaces. Another time for carb replenishment is following a workout. For immediate energy restoration and muscle building and mending, team carbs with a small serving of protein. (This safely replenishes muscle glycogen stores without the insulin rush and aids in fat burning.)

Later in the day opt for water-releasing carbs such as leafy green salads, broccoli, asparagus, and tomatoes. These have a high water content that keeps you hydrated during the night, plus they help cleanse your body of metabolic waste products.

You'll feel and look lighter day to day when you practice carbohydrate timing. The sample meal plans in the next chapter illustrate exactly how to put this strategy into practice.

Increase Your Postmeal Calorie Burn

After you eat a meal your body has to work to digest the food. In the process it burns some calories as body heat. This postmeal burn is technically known as thermogenesis, and it leads to an increase in your metabolism after eating. Studies of vegetarians reveal that they have a higher postmeal calorie burn than meat eaters do, so one way to boost your postmeal caloric burn is to consume lots of vegetables and fruits and keep your diet low in fat, as my Nutritional Life Plan recommends. By eating more plant foods and slashing the fat in your diet, you can keep your postmeal burn going for three or more hours after a meal.

Postmeal burn is partly due to insulin. Diets higher in plant foods improve your body's ability to use insulin, which ushers glucose into body cells for energy. This means it's easier to convert the nutrients you eat into fuel. In addition to the boost they give your metabolism after meals, plant-based diets also are lower in calories.

Eat Frequently Throughout the Day

To turn your body into a fat-melting furnace and keep your metabolism amped, try to eat every two to four hours, for a total of five or six meals a day. Every time you eat, your metabolism gets a boost due to thermogenesis, which I described on page 219. If you're eating frequently throughout the day, your metabolism will increase. Of course, a boosted metabolism is vital in your quest to lose fat.

A pattern of frequent eating keeps fat-forming cortisol in check too. When your body feels like it's spiraling down into starvation mode, as it does when you go on a crash diet, cortisol kicks in, and this can cause your body to retain fat, particularly around your middle.

Metabolically, frequent meals stabilize blood sugar levels and improve insulin release (elevated insulin levels inhibit fat burning), control appetite by taming hunger hormones, enhance glycogen storage so your body doesn't cannibalize metabolically active muscle, and keep your body's nutrient stores adequately supplied.

But remember, just because you're supposed to eat more frequently doesn't mean you should just eat anything in sight. You have to make sure you're choosing the right foods. Always be in control of what, when, and how much you eat.

Enjoy Healthy Snacks

One way to boost your eating frequency—and your metabolism—is to have healthy snacks. These include:

- Almonds and an apple or other fresh fruit
- Low-fat cheese stick with an orange
- Celery sticks or cucumber slices spread with hummus
- A vegetable serving such as celery with a teaspoon of almond or peanut butter
- Raw vegetables dipped in hummus
- Yogurt and fruit
- A fruit shake made with low-fat milk, whey protein, and fruit
- One cup of steamed edamame (soybeans) in the shell

Have Emergency Foods on Hand

I continually advise my clients to keep emergency foods with them. I came up with this strategy after seeing what happens when people get hungry and don't have healthy food around. They grab what's available—often something sweet, processed, and fattening.

That's why it's best to *always* have healthy food with you, *always*, wherever you go, whatever you do. When I travel, for example, I always pack my bag of almonds along with some fruit. That way I'm never subject to the peril of eating something that's not good for my metabolism or my health. It's all about planning and taking responsibility for what you eat. Don't let your meals plan you; *you* plan your meals.

Keep an Eye on Sodium

Loading up on salty foods, which are high in sodium, can throw your body off balance in ways you may not be aware of. Sodium works with another mineral, potassium, to maintain the correct balance of water in the body. The proper ratio of these two minerals helps prevent bloating (which results in weight gain), reduces blood pressure, and keeps your kidneys functioning normally. Too much sodium or too little potassium can upset this balance and create problems such as an irregular heartbeat and fatigue. When you're fatigued it affects your desire to exercise and, indirectly, your metabolism.

Expert opinions differ as to what is the correct ratio of potassium to sodium, but for optimum health it is generally thought to be 5 to 1 or even more. Most of us consume too much sodium and not enough potassium. Avoid salty and processed foods and increase your intake of fruits and vegetables (all loaded with potassium). Use nonsodium spices instead of salting your food and buy foods that marked "low-sodium."

Be Aware of Food Allergies

A potential cause of weight gain (mostly from water retention) and chronic bloatedness is food allergies or food sensitivities. A food allergy is an abnormal response to a food by your immune system. (A food sensitivity is also an abnormal response to food, but it does not affect the immune system.) Normally your immune system helps defend your body against harmful bacteria and viruses, but sometimes it identifies certain foods as harmful, triggering an allergic reaction. Usually the protein in a food causes the reaction, which may show up as one or more of the following:

- Weight gain. You may gain an excessive amount of water weight as your body tries to dilute the allergen.
- Bloatedness, particularly in the abdominal area.
- A tingling sensation in your mouth and swelling of your lips.
- Cramping, nausea, vomiting, and diarrhea.
- Hives and itching.
- Wheezing, shortness of breath, and a stuffy nose.
- Dizziness or light-headedness.

221

A few foods are responsible for most people's allergies and sensitivities. Peanuts, tree nuts such as walnuts and almonds, fish, and shellfish are the biggest culprits for adults.

Another common sensitivity is to gluten, a protein found in bread flour. Gluten causes bread to rise when it is leavened with yeast. Whole grains such as wheat, oats, rye, buckwheat, and barley also contain gluten (corn, rice, millet, soybean, and peanut flour do not). Commercial baked foods are full of gluten. Many people simply cannot digest gluten, and if they eat it, may experience a bloated abdomen, diarrhea, muscle wasting (bad for your metabolism!), loss of appetite, gas, digestive pain, and serious malnutrition because many of these symptoms cause loss of nutrients. I am one of those people who contend with gluten intolerance. After eating certain breads, for example, I have abdominal distention, gas, and general discomfort. So I've really cut back on breads and other gluten-containing foods. Fortunately there are many gluten-free products on the market, so you do not have to deprive yourself if you have this particular food sensitivity. Your physician can help you identify whether you have a sensitivity to gluten (or other foods); if you do, it's easy to adjust your diet and lifestyle so gluten does not intrude on your health.

Be on the alert too, for foods containing high-fructose corn syrup, a low-cost additive found in many foods. Six times sweeter than sugar, it helps prevent frozen foods from developing freezer burn and keeps packaged foods soft and fresh-tasting longer. Many people can't properly digest this additive, and the malabsorption leads to the release of hydrogen gas, causing diarrhea, abdominal pain, and bloating.

The body metabolizes concentrated fructose differently from sugar, more easily converting it into fat. The conversion may also raise levels of triglycerides, which are implicated in heart disease. Avoiding high-fructose corn syrup may help you lose excess weight and improve your overall health. Start by eliminating processed foods and sodas from your diet. And read food labels! If high-fructose corn syrup is one of the top ingredients on the label, put the item back on the shelf.

Use Smart Sweeteners

I'm not such a purist that I'm against artificial sweeteners. They do have their place when you like a touch of sweetness in your coffee or sprinkled on foods. There's certainly nothing wrong with the occasional use of small amounts of artificial sweeteners.

There are now more artificial sweeteners on the market than ever, so it's challenging to figure out which ones are best. I recommend xylitol, sold as Perfect Sweet, Miracle Sweet, and Health Sweet in the United States. Xylitol is a sugar alcohol that has been used in diabetic foods for many years. These days sugar alcohols are appearing in many nondiabetic foods. They are digested slowly and don't raise blood sugar as rapidly as sugar does, so they have a minimal effect on blood sugar and insulin. If you ingest too much, though, you can experience bloating, gas, and diarrhea, because sugar alcohols travel unabsorbed through the intestinal tract.

Like most sugar alcohols, xylitol is as bulky as sugar, so you can use it tablespoon for tablespoon to replace sugar in recipes. You can also cook with sugar alcohols.

Stay Hydrated

Water is the ultimate beverage for your metabolism. It can't be overemphasized. Emerging research shows that water may play an important role in regulating your metabolism. If you become dehydrated—that is, low on water—your metabolism may slow to a crawl. Of course that means you won't burn as much fat or as many calories. Dehydration also leads to fatigue and low energy; under those conditions you cannot give your workouts your best levels of intensity, and consequently, you won't develop fat-burning muscle as efficiently or as effectively. You need sufficient water to help dilute, dissolve, and eliminate toxins that can otherwise interfere with muscle recovery and development.

How much water should you drink while following my Nutritional Life Plan? My recommendation is *eight to ten 8-ounce glasses* a day. If you don't like plain water, try some of the fitness waters on the market or the bottled waters that are lightly flavored without calories and sugars. You can also squeeze some lemon or lime juice into plain water.

As long as you get your eight to 10 glasses of water in a day, you may drink other beverages too, such as diet decaffeinated sodas and herbal teas.

If you drink coffee, cut your intake to a minimum (1 cup per day). As you know, coffee contains caffeine, and caffeine makes you store fat by hiking cortisol levels. Green tea is the caffeinated drink of choice because it has well-known antioxidant and metabolic benefits, plus ample amounts of water. I strongly recommend a minimum of 1–2 cups of green tea (preferably decaf) per day. Green tea helps greatly in eliminating any water retention issues as well. You can track your daily consumption of green tea in your *Make Over Your Metabolism* food journal on page 225.

What About Alcohol?

I'm glad you asked! If you want to occasionally enjoy some alcohol, choose red wine—it is high in the following disease-fighting antioxidants.

- Saponins, which appear to reduce the risk of cardiovascular disease by preventing the absorption of cholesterol in the body.
- Resveratrol, which offers some cardiovascular benefits and may inhibit tumor development in some cancers. It may also aid in the formation of nerve cells, protecting against diseases like Alzheimer's and Parkinson's down the road.
- Polyphenols, which strongly inhibit the chemicals that make blood vessels constrict, thereby reducing the number of fatty streaks in the vessels and decreasing the risk of heart attack.

A red flag warning here: The health benefits of red wine are still being studied and debated in research circles. While the jury is still out, you can enjoy an occasional glass of wine as long as you're not prone to alcoholism and there aren't any other reasons alcohol could have an negative impact on your health and your life. Keep in mind that moderation is key.

Keep It Real

The best nutritional advice I can leave you with is to eat foods in as close to their natural state as possible. That means selecting fresh fruits and vegetables, whole grains, lean proteins, and thin fats like the ones I've mentioned. We need to get back to natural wholesome foods and hustle overly processed foods out of our diet. Eating right isn't really all that complicated if you stick to real food—and stop obsessing over food pyramids and carb counting. Eat real food that you prepare and cook yourself. Remember: Real food rocks!

Make Over Your Metabolism
Food Journal

Date _____ Day of the Week _____

Breakfast: Time I ate _____

Foods I ate _____

_____

This meal included: ☐ Protein ☐ Carbs ☐ Fat ☐ Fiber (g)_____

Mid-Morning Snack: Time I ate _____

Foods I ate _____

This meal included: ☐ Protein ☐ Carbs ☐ Fat ☐ Fiber (g)

Lunch: Time I ate _____

Foods I ate _____

_____

This meal included: ☐ Protein ☐ Carbs ☐ Fat ☐ Fiber (g)_____

Mid-Afternoon Snack: Time I ate _____

Foods I ate _____

This meal included: ☐ Protein ☐ Carbs ☐ Fat ☐ Fiber (g)_____

Dinner: Time I ate _____

Foods I ate _____

_____

This meal included: ☐ Protein ☐ Carbs ☐ Fat ☐ Fiber (g)_____

Total 8-ounce glasses of water I had today _____ Total cups of green tea I had today _____

Did you follow the Nutritional Life Plan today? **Yes No**

If not, what do I need to work on tomorrow?_____

Did you get your protein at 4 of the 5 meals? **Yes No**

Did you get your 25–50 grams of fiber today? **Yes No**

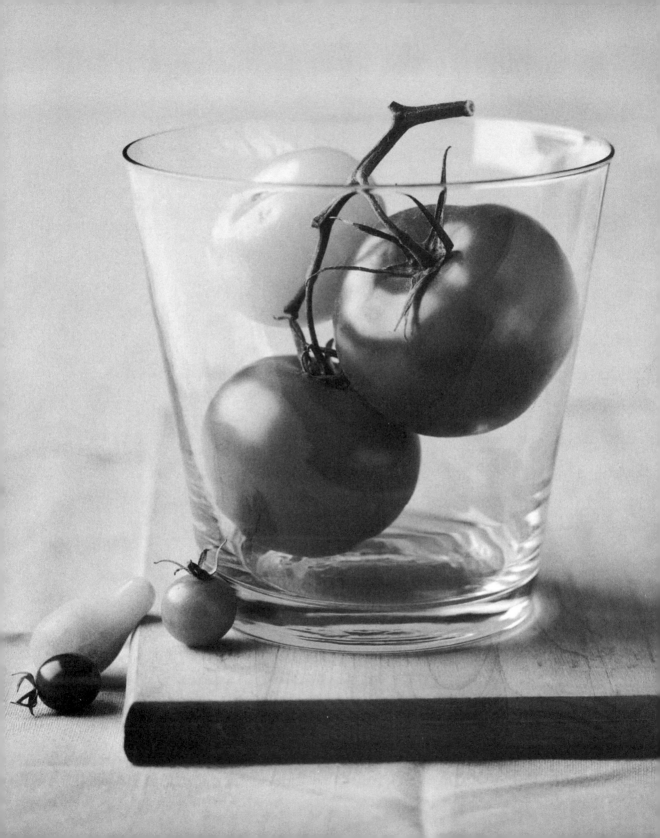

Chapter Nine

THE PLAN YOU ARE ABOUT TO FOLLOW FOCUSES ON LOSING BODY FAT, BUT AT THE SAME TIME, IT HELPS YOU MAKE SMALL YET VERY HEALTHY ALTERATIONS TO YOUR LIFESTYLE. THERE ARE NO GIMMICKS HERE. IF YOU HAVE EVER FOLLOWED a weight-loss diet, you know that gimmicks don't work. Sure you may lose weight on a fad diet, but I'm willing to bet the weight will return. The truth is that to lose body fat, get fit, and rev up your metabolism, you need an approach to eating that you can live with for the rest of your life. This is it.

A few preliminaries:

- **Eat five times daily:** breakfast, lunch, dinner, and two snacks.
- **Eat protein at four of the five meals.**
- **Enjoy one or two servings of lean beef a week.**
- **Have several weekly servings of coldwater fish,** such as salmon, tuna, halibut, mackerel, and herring. These protein foods are loaded with omega-3 fatty acids, which have an array of health benefits. I also recommend

4 Weeks to Healthy, Get-Fit Eating

sushi, if it's available in your area. Order it with brown rice or some cooked greens for a very complete and healthy meal.

- **Include game meats as part of your protein choices,** if you so desire. They are low in fat, low in cholesterol, and high in protein—and they're the original organic alternative. The American Heart Association recommends venison, rabbit, pheasant, and duck (without skin) as low-fat alternatives to typical meats.

- **Eat two servings a day of fresh fruit for the first 14 days.** After that have three daily servings of fruit.

- **Enjoy unlimited amounts of raw or steamed nonstarchy vegetables every day.** Concentrate on water-releasing vegetables, such as asparagus, cucumbers, and greens.

- **Eliminate starches at dinner, unless you've had a particularly active day.** Avoiding these carbs at night—and focusing on the nonstarchy carbs—leads to speedier fat loss. By all means, though, have a starch at breakfast and lunch.

- **Drink one or two cups of decaffeinated green tea every day.** Green tea contains valuable antioxidants, plus natural chemicals that enhance your metabolism and help your body burn fat. Not only that, green tea actually helps your insulin regulate your blood sugar more effectively. And again, it helps in a big way to curb water retention. Record the number of cups of green tea consumed per day in your food journal.

- **Use spices liberally, and with imagination, to flavor your foods.** Try lemon, garlic, pepper, Italian spices, and so forth. Cayenne pepper is a good choice because research has shown that it boosts metabolism.

- **Flavor your food with vinegar and lemon juice and choose salad dressings containing vinegar and lemon juice.** These condiments create reductions in insulin responses, and this is metabolically favorable to weight control.

- **Stay hydrated.** Make sure you drink eight to ten 8-ounce glasses of pure water daily, a good habit that enhances your metabolism.

Learn to Take Control of Your Food—No Matter What the Situation

As you apply the Nutritional Life Plan to your own life, you'll be taking control of what you eat, no matter where you go or what you do. Plan your meals as you plan your business meetings or a church or charity function. Plan, plan, and plan. Always have your emergency foods with you as well so that you never have to be tempted by the food around you. As you plan your life, plan the essence of life, which is food.

If you go to a restaurant, have the mind-set that you are cooking the same food at home. You've got to take control as if you were at home. I've worked in a restaurant before, and I've seen chefs toss in vats of butter, fat, and sodium to make food taste better. Would you cook with a vatful of grease? No. So look at the menu carefully and ask for alternatives. If you're not sure what's in the sauce or the dressing, have it on the side. Similarly, ask that vegetables be steamed and meats be grilled without added fat. Tell them what you want. After all, you are the customer, and the restaurant wants your business!

This goes for fast food restaurants too. To save calories, carbohydrates, and some gluten, have a sandwich with only part of the bun. Don't be shy about telling the server to eliminate the mayonnaise, the special sauce, or the cheese. Or forget the sandwich and order a salad instead. There are plenty of ways to take control of your choices, even at fast-food establishments.

Before you go grocery shopping, take time to eat so you won't be hungry and make unhealthy impulse purchases. Always take a list with you to the store so you'll stay focused on buying the healthy foods you need. To make your list, plan the meals you want to prepare for the next few days, check around your kitchen to see what you have on hand, and write down the ingredients you need.

Once in the grocery store, keep in mind that the healthiest foods, such as fresh produce and unprocessed meats, tend to be placed around the perimeter of the store. Stay clear, for the most part, of the center aisles. That's where all the high-calorie processed foods—and everything that's usually loaded with sodium and additives—are shelved.

Parties are another potential war zone in your battle to control unhealthy impulse eating. Take control! Make the healthiest choices you can. If you're attending a company function, don't be afraid to bring your emergency food along. Or eat before you go so you won't give in to temptation. If you're at a cocktail party and don't want to drink a lot of alcohol, grab a carbonated water or club soda, put a lime in it, and it will look just like a gin and tonic.

229

Taking control extends to what your family eats too. There's no reason your family can't adopt good eating habits also. Have healthy snacks on hand for munching—fruits, low-fat or nonfat cheeses, almonds, vegetables, lean turkey, and so forth. This will help curtail a lot of the junk food and sugar kids especially tend to eat.

In the table below you'll see comparisons of unhealthy and healthy meals (without snacks included). Think about the consequences of your eating choices. Is indulgence worth the weight gain over time? The next time you reach for something that's not on the Nutritional Life Plan, think about how unhealthy choices can really add up in terms of fat pounds.

	Unhealthy Meals			Healthy Meals	
Breakfast	Lunch	**Dinner**	Breakfast	**Lunch**	Dinner
3 fried eggs	Fast-food cheese-burger	**8-ounce prime rib**	2 egg whites, scrambled	**Large salad topped with tuna and olive oil vinaigrette**	4-ounce round steak
3 bacon strips	Medium order of fries	**Baked potato with sour cream and butter**	3 lean turkey bacon strips		Steamed green beans (1 cup)
1 biscuit with pat of butter	12-ounce cola	**Salad with blue cheese dressing**	1 slice whole grain toast	**Baked potato, plain**	Chopped fresh fruit for dessert (1 cup)
Glass of orange juice (8 ounces)		**Large piece of dinner bread with pat of butter**	½ grapefruit		
Coffee with cream		**Piece of cheesecake for dessert**	Decaf green tea (1 cup)		
Calories: 685	Calories: 952	**Calories: 1,440**	Calories: 265	**Calories: 435**	Calories: 326
Total Daily Calories: 3,077			Total Daily Calories: 1,026		

Lose Weight for Good

Please remember that this isn't a diet. Nor are the exercise routines a temporary fix. They are meant to be lifestyle changes—a life plan for keeping your metabolism in good working order indefinitely. The *Make Over Your Metabolism* program gets easier the longer you stick to it. You'll begin to love eating delicious healthy food five times a day. You'll love the way your body looks and feels. You'll end your love-hate relationship with food and exercise because you've learned how to sustain automatic fat burn 24-7.

I hope you are beginning to see how easy losing weight, fat, and inches can be if you follow the *Make Over Your Metabolism* program. These metabolism-boosting changes can stay with you forever. You'll gain energy, and you'll be more protected against many serious diseases. Oh, did I mention that you'll begin to look and feel younger too?

My hope is that this program will serve as your road map to a new lifestyle. Sure, sometimes you'll stray off course. It's normal. Don't obsess or worry about it or punish yourself. Just take responsibility. But if you really want to reach your destination, you've got to look at the map and get back on the right road. You're in the driver's seat of your life, and now you have directions you can follow for the rest of your life. Make it the best journey you can!

If you consume daily ...*	Expect to gain this much weight in a year's time
Two 12-ounce soft drinks ...	**31 pounds**
1 glazed doughnut ...	21 pounds
1 large muffin ...	**33 pounds**
1 large latte with whole milk ...	35 pounds
1 chocolate candy bar ...	**24 pounds**
1 serving of potato chips ...	17 pounds
1 medium order of french fries ...	**46 pounds**
1 cup of ice cream ...	59 pounds

*This information is based on common calorie counts of the foods listed. Results vary from person to person. Annual weight gain is based on the yearly caloric total divided by 3,500 (the number of calories it takes to gain 1 pound of fat).

Nutritional Life Plan Menus

DAY 1—MONDAY

Breakfast

1 egg
> poached, hard- or soft-boiled, scrambled, or pan-cooked with 1 teaspoon of "light" canola or olive oil to coat the pan

1 cup All-Bran cereal with ½ cup nonfat milk

½ cup boysenberries

1 cup green tea (preferred) or coffee

Morning snack

1 orange

Lunch

Chicken breast

Small salad with 1 tablespoon light olive oil vinaigrette or nonfat dressing

⅓ cup cooked brown rice

½ cup blueberries

Water

Afternoon snack

8–10 almonds (no salt)

Celery sticks

1 cup decaffeinated green tea

Dinner

Salmon, filet or canned

1 cup steamed broccoli

4 slices fresh tomato with balsamic vinegar

Water

DAY 2—TUESDAY

Breakfast

2 small light, low-sodium (organic preferred) turkey sausage links

1 cup whole grain oatmeal

½ cup raspberries

1 cup green tea (preferred) or coffee

Morning snack

1 apple

Lunch

Tuna over salad greens and chopped vegetables with 1 tablespoon light olive oil vinaigrette or nonfat dressing

½ cup mixed legumes or legume of choice

Water

Afternoon snack

Celery sticks spread with 1 tablespoon of hummus

1 cup decaffeinated green tea

Dinner

Grilled lamb chop

1 cup steamed cauliflower (mashed, if you desire)

Sliced cucumber

Water

Note: Even though there are quantities for vegetables listed each day, you can eat them in unlimited quantities.

DAY 3—WEDNESDAY

Breakfast
Whole grain toast spread with 1 teaspoon
    peanut or almond butter
1 peach
½ cup nonfat milk
1 cup green tea (preferred) or coffee

Morning snack
1 cup cottage cheese with choice of
    fresh berries

Lunch
Grilled top-grade "lean" beef choice
½ cup cooked quinoa
Sliced tomatoes
Water

Afternoon snack
Carrot or zucchini sticks
5 almonds (no salt)
1 cup decaffeinated green tea

Dinner
Grilled tilapia or other whitefish
1 cup steamed cabbage
5 asparagus spears
Water

DAY 4—THURSDAY

Breakfast
1 egg
    poached, hard- or soft-boiled, scrambled,
    or pan-cooked with 1 teaspoon of "light"
    canola or olive oil to coat the pan
1 cup whole grain hot cereal
½ cantaloupe
1 cup green tea (preferred) or coffee

Morning snack
5–10 almonds (no salt)
1 cup choice of fresh berries

Lunch
Small Cobb salad of lettuce, turkey,
    tomatoes, and egg with 1 tablespoon
    olive oil vinaigrette or nonfat dressing
Water

Afternoon snack
1 cup sugar-free yogurt
1 cup decaffeinated green tea

Dinner
Baked chicken breast
1 cup steamed spinach
1 cup Brussels sprouts
Water

DAY 5—FRIDAY

Breakfast
2 small links low-fat chicken sausage
1 cup high-fiber cereal with
    ½ cup nonfat milk
1 cup choice of fresh berries
1 cup green tea (preferred) or coffee

Morning snack
1 orange
4-5 walnuts (plain)

Lunch
Turkey wrap
    with 1 whole wheat pita or tortilla,
    lettuce, tomato, ⅛ slice avocado, and
    1 tablespoon nonfat mayonnaise or nonfat
    plain yogurt
Water

Afternoon snack
Raw veggie sticks of choice
1 cup decaffeinated green tea

Dinner
Grilled salmon fillet
1 cup green beans
Cucumber slices
Water

DAY 6—SATURDAY

Breakfast
Whey protein shake
    made with 1 banana, 2 scoops whey
    protein mix, 1 cup nonfat milk, ice, and
    ½ cup blueberries
1 cup green tea (preferred) or coffee

Morning snack
5–10 almonds (no salt)
2 fresh mango slices

Lunch
3 or 4 medium-size steamed shrimp
½ cup couscous
Small green salad with 1 tablespoon
    vinaigrette or nonfat dressing
Water

Afternoon snack
⅔ cup legumes of choice
1 cup decaffeinated green tea

Dinner
Grilled halibut with garlic
Steamed bell pepper
3 or 4 slices fresh tomato
Water

DAY 7—SUNDAY

Breakfast
1 egg
poached, hard- or soft-boiled, scrambled,
or pan-cooked with 1 teaspoon of "light"
canola or olive oil to coat the pan
1 cup cooked buckwheat
½ grapefruit
1 cup green tea (preferred) or coffee

Morning snack
1 honeydew melon wedge
1 teaspoon hummus

Lunch
Small grilled chicken burger lettuce wrap
with tomato, sprouts, lettuce, and nonfat
mozzarella cheese
½ cup cooked millet
Water

Afternoon snack
2 fresh apricots
1 cup decaffeinated green tea

Dinner
Grilled shark or tuna steak
1 cup steamed broccoli
1 cup steamed cauliflower
Water

DAY 8—MONDAY

Breakfast
2 turkey or chicken sausage links (low-sodium
and organic preferred)
1 cup high-fiber oatmeal
1 wedge cantaloupe
1 cup green tea (preferred) or coffee

Morning snack
1 cup sugar-free yogurt

Lunch
Grilled lean hamburger
½ cup cooked quinoa
5 or 6 asparagus spears
Water

Afternoon snack
1 apple
5–10 almonds (no salt)
1 cup decaffeinated green tea

Dinner
Grilled haddock
Small green salad with 1 tablespoon olive oil
vinaigrette or nonfat dressing
1 cup cooked dandelion or other greens
Water

DAY 9—TUESDAY

Breakfast
One egg
poached, hard- or soft-boiled, scrambled,
or pan-cooked with a teaspoon of light
canola or olive oil to coat the pan
1 cup high-fiber cereal with
½ cup nonfat milk
Pineapple slice (fresh or canned in its own
juice with no added sugar)
1 cup green tea (preferred) or coffee

Morning snack
Celery sticks spread with 1 tablespoon
peanut butter

Lunch
Grilled chicken breast
Baked sweet potato or yam (with the skin)
½ cup cooked turnip greens
Water

Afternoon snack
1 cup choice of fresh fruit
1 cup decaffeinated green tea

Dinner
Grilled lamb chop with chopped garlic
1 cup steamed green beans and bok choy
3 slices fresh tomato
Water

DAY 10—WEDNESDAY

Breakfast
1 slice whole grain toast with 1 teaspoon
peanut or almond butter
1 cup fresh berries
1 cup green tea (preferred) or coffee

Morning snack
1 cup low-fat cottage cheese
1 piece fresh fruit or ½ cup fresh berries

Lunch
Tuna lettuce wrap
with tomato, sprouts, and 1 tablespoon
light grated Parmesan cheese with a
low-carb tortilla
Water

Afternoon snack
Celery, zucchini, or cucumber slices
1 cup decaffeinated green tea

Dinner
Baked turkey breast
1 cup steamed Brussels sprouts
½ steamed bell pepper
Water

DAY 11—THURSDAY

Breakfast
2 egg whites, scrambled
½ cup cooked bulgur with ¼ cup cranberries
1 cup green tea (preferred) or coffee

Morning snack
1 slice low-fat feta cheese
1 orange

Lunch
Grilled chicken burger
Small green salad with 1 tablespoon olive oil
    vinaigrette or nonfat dressing
Carrot sticks
Water

Afternoon snack
5–10 almonds (no salt)
1 slice of pineapple (fresh or canned in its
    own juice with no sugar added)
1 cup decaffeinated green tea

Dinner
Grilled salmon with garlic
Parsley
Steamed broccoli with lemon and
    pepper spices
Water

DAY 12—FRIDAY

Breakfast
Whey protein shake
    made with 1 banana, 2 scoops whey
    protein mix, 1 cup nonfat milk, ice, and
    ½ cup blueberries

Morning snack
5 ounces fresh pomegranate juice
5–10 almonds (no salt)

Lunch
Grilled orange roughy
½ cup summer squash
1 cup mustard greens or greens of choice
Water

Afternoon snack
Cucumber and zucchini slices
1 cup decaffeinated green tea

Dinner
Baked Cornish game hen
1 cup steamed watercress
1 cup steamed Brussels sprouts
Water

DAY 13—SATURDAY

Breakfast
One egg
    poached, hard- or soft-boiled, scrambled,
    or pan-cooked with a teaspoon of light
    canola or olive oil to coat the pan
1 cup bran cereal with ½ cup nonfat milk
1 honeydew melon wedge
1 cup green tea (preferred) or coffee

Morning snack
4 carrot sticks dipped in hummus

Lunch
Turkey lettuce wrap
    with tomato, sprouts, and 1 tablespoon
    light grated Parmesan cheese with a low-
    carb tortilla
Water

Afternoon snack
1 apple or orange
5–10 almonds (no salt)
1 cup decaffeinated green tea

Dinner
Grilled shrimp with grilled onions
Small green salad with 1 tablespoon olive oil
    vinaigrette or nonfat dressing
Water

DAY 14—SUNDAY

Breakfast
2 small links chicken or turkey sausage
    (low-sodium and organic preferred)
1 slice whole grain toast
½ cup blueberries
1 cup green tea (preferred) or coffee

Morning snack
1 tangerine
1 slice nonfat mozzarella cheese

Lunch
Grilled red snapper
½ cup combo of red and garbanzo beans
1 cup steamed broccoli
Water

Afternoon snack
Celery sticks
5–10 almonds or walnuts (no salt)
1 cup decaffeinated green tea

Dinner
Grilled trout with lemon and garlic
1 cup steamed cabbage with scallions
½ cup steamed mushrooms
Water

DAY 15—MONDAY

Breakfast
Grilled tofu steak
1 cup bran oatmeal
Orange slices
1 cup green tea (preferred) or coffee

Morning snack
5–10 almonds (no salt)
1 peach

Lunch
Grilled lean hamburger or beef portion
Steamed asparagus
½ cup steamed summer squash
Water

Afternoon snack
1 apple
1 cup decaffeinated green tea

Dinner
Grilled salmon fillet (canned in water)
    or halibut
1 cup steamed red cabbage
1 cup steamed zucchini
Water

DAY 16—TUESDAY

Breakfast
2 egg whites, scrambled
1 cup bran cereal with ½ cup nonfat milk
1 slice pineapple (fresh or canned in its own
    juice with no sugar added)
1 cup green tea (preferred) or coffee

Morning snack
1 cup sugar-free yogurt

Lunch
Grilled sole
⅓ cup whole wheat or gluten-free pasta
1 cup broccoli steamed with garlic cloves
Water

Afternoon snack
Celery sticks
5–10 almonds or walnuts (no salt)
1 cup decaffeinated green tea

Dinner
Baked turkey stuffed with spinach
1 cup Brussels sprouts with watercress
Water

DAY 17—WEDNESDAY

Breakfast
1 cup cottage cheese
1 slice whole grain toast
½ cup fresh berries of choice
1 cup green tea (preferred) or coffee

Morning snack
½ cup legumes of choice with balsamic
     vinegar

Lunch
Chicken lettuce wrap
     with tomato, sprouts, lettuce, and
     chopped or mashed fresh garlic
Water

Afternoon snack
1 peach
8-10 almonds or walnuts (no salt)
1 cup decaffeinated green tea

Dinner
Chicken breast, baked with grapes
1 cup steamed cauliflower
Small green salad with radishes and
     1 tablespoon light olive oil vinaigrette or
     nonfat dressing
Water

DAY 18—THURSDAY

Breakfast
2 egg whites, scrambled
1 cup bran cereal with ½ cup nonfat milk
½ pear
1 cup green tea (preferred) or coffee

Morning snack
Celery or zucchini sticks
1 teaspoon peanut or almond butter

Lunch
Grilled swordfish or shark
½ baked potato with skin with
     1 teaspoon olive oil drizzled on top
1 cup steamed kale
Water

Afternoon snack
1 plum
1 cup decaffeinated green tea

Dinner
Chicken slices baked with snow peas
1 cup steamed Brussels sprouts
Water

DAY 19—FRIDAY

Breakfast
Omelet of 3 egg whites with spinach and
    scallions
½ cup fresh berries of choice
1 cup green tea (preferred) or coffee

Morning snack
½ cup mashed black and red beans with
    carrot sticks for dipping

Lunch
Grilled tofu steak
½ cup wild and brown rice mixture
1 cup steamed broccoli
Water

Afternoon snack
Peach, apricot, apple, or orange
1 cup decaffeinated green tea

Dinner
Grilled sirloin (ultralean) with onions
    and garlic
1 cup steamed cabbage, red and green
Water

DAY 20—SATURDAY

Breakfast
Whey protein shake
    made with 1 banana, 2 scoops whey
    protein mix, 1 cup nonfat milk, ice, and
    8-10 blueberries
1 cup green tea (preferred) or coffee

Morning snack
Celery sticks spread with 1 teaspoon hummus

Lunch
Grilled chicken breast with garlic
Baked yam or sweet potato with skin
½ cup kale
Water

Afternoon snack
Green-skin apple
1 cup decaffeinated green tea

Dinner
Grilled tuna steak
1 cup dandelion greens or other greens
5 or 6 asparagus spears
Water

DAY 21—SUNDAY

Breakfast
2 small chicken or turkey sausage links
    (low-sodium and organic preferred)
1 cup bran oatmeal
½ cup raspberries
1 cup green tea (preferred) or coffee

Morning snack
5-10 almonds (no salt)
1 honeydew melon wedge

Lunch
Grilled tilapia or other whitefish
½ cup black beans with onions
1 cup steamed broccoli
Water

Afternoon snack
1 slice nonfat mozzarella cheese
Veggie sticks
1 cup decaffeinated green tea

Dinner
Baked lamb loin steak
1 cup steamed collard greens
Arugula salad with 1 teaspoon olive oil
    vinaigrette
Water

DAY 22—MONDAY

Breakfast
2 egg whites, scrambled
1 slice whole grain toast
1 cup raspberries
1 cup green tea (preferred) or coffee

Morning snack
1 cup nonfat yogurt with ½ fresh peach

Lunch
Turkey or chicken lettuce wrap
    with tomato, sprouts, and light Parmesan
    cheese
½ cup blueberries
Water

Afternoon snack
½ cup legumes of choice
1 cup decaffeinated green tea

Dinner
Grilled salmon with garlic and lemon
1 cup steamed mashed cauliflower
1 cup dandelion greens or greens of choice
Water

DAY 23—TUESDAY

Breakfast
1 grilled tofu steak
1 cup bran cereal with ½ cup nonfat milk
½ cantaloupe
1 cup green tea (preferred) or coffee

Morning snack
1 slice nonfat mozzarella cheese
1 orange

Lunch
Grilled beef burger or sirloin (ultralean)
½ cup summer squash
1 cup steamed broccoli
Water

Afternoon snack
1 cup mixed berries
1 cup decaffeinated green tea

Dinner
Grilled trout with lemon, onion, and garlic
1 cup steamed zucchini
1 cup steamed cabbage
Water

DAY 24—WEDNESDAY

Breakfast
1 breakfast chicken sausage patty (low-sodium
      and organic preferred)
1 cup nonfat yogurt with 1 cup boysenberries
1 cup green tea (preferred) or coffee

Morning snack
½ cup legume mixture prepared in
      food processor
Carrot or zucchini sticks for dipping

Lunch
Turkey wrap
      with whole grain tortilla, tomatoes,
      lettuce, fresh garlic, and sprouts
Water

Afternoon snack
1 apple
1 cup decaffeinated green tea

Dinner
Grilled lamb chop
1 cup steamed green beans
Small green salad with 1 tablespoon olive oil
      vinaigrette or nonfat dressing
Water

DAY 25—THURSDAY

Breakfast
2 turkey bacon slices (no nitrates)
1 cup bran cereal with ½ cup nonfat milk
½ cup blueberries
1 cup green tea (preferred) or coffee

Morning snack
Cucumber and carrot slices dipped in
1 tablespoon hummus

Lunch
Grilled chicken breast
Small green salad with 1 tablespoon olive oil
vinaigrette
1 cup steamed okra
Water

Afternoon snack
1 pear
5–10 almonds (no salt)
1 cup decaffeinated green tea

Dinner
Steamed clams with lemon, pepper, onion,
and garlic
10 spears steamed asparagus
Water

DAY 26—FRIDAY

Breakfast
1 egg and 1 egg white scrambled with onions
and peppers
1 slice Ezekiel bread toast
½ cup raspberries
1 cup green tea (preferred) or coffee

Morning snack
1 cup sugar-free yogurt with ½ sliced banana

Lunch
Grilled cod
½ baked potato with skin with 1 teaspoon
olive oil drizzled on top
1 cup cucumber salad with balsamic
vinegar only
Water

Afternoon snack
5-10 almonds (no salt)
1 apple
1 cup decaffeinated green tea

Dinner
Baked turkey breast with garlic and spinach
Small green salad with nonfat dressing
Water

DAY 27—SATURDAY

Breakfast

1 slice whole grain toast with 1 teaspoon
    almond butter or peanut butter
1 cup blueberries and raspberries mixed
1 cup green tea (preferred) or coffee

Morning snack

Celery and cucumber slices
1 slice nonfat mozzarella cheese

Lunch

Grilled salmon with garlic and lemon
½ cup black beans
1 cup alfalfa sprouts
Water

Afternoon snack

1 orange
1 cup decaffeinated green tea

Dinner

Baked Cornish game hen with onions and
    dandelion greens
Small green salad with nonfat dressing or
    olive oil vinaigrette
Water

DAY 28—SUNDAY

Breakfast

2 egg whites, scrambled
1 cup bran cereal with ½ cup nonfat milk
½ banana
1 cup green tea (preferred) or coffee

Morning snack

½ cup cottage cheese with 2 slices pineapple
    (fresh or canned in its own juice with no
    sugar added)

Lunch

Steamed crab
½ cup brown rice and wild rice mixture
5 or 6 steamed asparagus spears
Water

Afternoon snack

Cucumber slices
¼ cup red and garbanzo beans, mixed
1 cup decaffeinated green tea

Dinner

Grilled chicken breast
1 cup steamed broccoli
1 cup steamed cabbage
Water

Appendix

Robert's Rules for Creating a Home Gym to Suit Your Budget, Space, and Goals

I've talked to you about working out at home and have given you many options for doing so. Now I'd like to offer further guidance on setting up a home fitness facility that will meet all your exercise needs.

Shop for Equipment

For starters, where should you go to buy exercise equipment? Begin at your nearest fitness specialty store. These stores focus on fitness equipment and accessories, and they'll have a wide array of choices. Most likely there will be staff members who were hired because they are fitness enthusiasts; they can guide you in the right direction. If there is no fitness specialty store in your area, try the fitness department in your local sporting goods store. Department stores also have sections dedicated to sports and fitness. Do your homework before you go to the store. Know your fitness goals, your abilities, and the activities you enjoy or have had success with in the past. Talk to your doctor. Ask questions of the person at the store. Make well-thought-out decisions about your equipment choices. This should not be impulse buying.

Some infomercials do sell products that are very worthwhile and should be considered for your home gym. However, before you whip out your credit card and dial the 800 number, do some research. Search the Internet for fitness and exercise equipment. Consult consumer guides. Pay a visit to your YMCA. These public fitness centers have the best equipment to lure and maintain paying members. Spend a little time at one of these facilities and try different modes of exercise. This is a great trial ground for products you may want to include in your home facility. Call the manufacturer of a product you are interested in to get more information. Shop as though you were buying a car! You want to know if the equipment you are purchasing is right for you. You will be spending a great deal of time with your exercise equipment in what you hope will be a long-term relationship. Here are some questions to think about when evaluating equipment for your home gym:

- What are you actually doing on the equipment?
- Is the motion comfortable for you?
- Does the product provide you with an activity that you enjoy?
- Is it safe?
- Is the product sturdy? What is it made of?
- Will it fit in the space you have allotted?
- Is there a warranty or service available in the event of a breakdown?
- If you cannot move the equipment on your own, is there delivery and expert setup available?

Consult with a Health Care Professional

Among the most important and reliable sources of information about what products to put in your home workout facility are your doctor, chiropractor, and physical therapist. They should know your capabilities and limitations. Talk to them about exercises or physical activity that you have enjoyed and were successful in doing in the past. In most cases these practitioners will be up on current exercise systems and can offer insights to guide you in the right direction.

Ask for a 30-Day Return Policy

I cannot emphasize enough: Whatever you buy, be it a jump rope or a four-stack multi-station gym, make absolutely sure you have a 30-day trial period in which to use the product in your home. Try the product right away to get the full feel of the exercise so you can decide whether the equipment is right for you. Most specialty stores, sporting goods stores, and major retailers will provide this policy. If you don't like what you bought and it will not help you stay consistent in meeting your fitness goals, exchange it for something that does meet your needs.

It is your loss if you pass the 30-day point and you discover that what you have purchased does not meet your needs. If you do not take advantage of this time period, you may be stuck with yet another dust collector or place to hang the laundry.

Consider This Equipment

These are some of the equipment choices I recommend to my clients who work out at their homes:

- Elliptical trainer with or without arm motion (see page 79)
- Treadmill
- Stepping machine
- Multistation home gym
- Step mill
- Ski machine
- Lateral slide kit
- Upright stationary bike
- Recumbent stationary bike with or without arm motion
- Swimming weights
- Rowing machine

The following equipment, most of which you can see in my exercise demonstration photographs throughout *Make Over Your Metabolism,* is available online at www.robertreames.net.

- Tubing/exercise bands
- Dumbbells
- Stability balls
- Medicine balls
- Exercise mats
- Jump ropes
- Pedometers
- Step-up units (pictured this page)

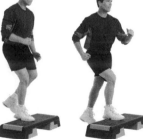

- The Stick
- Deluxe Exerciser
- Workout bench
- Heart rate monitors

A note on multistation gyms: These are the units that you see in commercial fitness centers, YMCAs, apartment complexes, schools, and recreation centers. They provide a variety of exercise options in one unit with several stations working off of a single weight stack or multiple weight stacks. More weight stacks mean more than one person can work with the unit at a time. Multistation gyms provide exercises for your entire body. They are safe and, in most cases, very simple to operate.

Before purchasing, compare the structure and strength of the units for sale. Structure is based on the gauge of steel used, the tensile strength of the cables, and quality of the pulleys. If you can shake the unit excessively in the store, chances are it's not very stable. I recommend buying your multistation gym at a specialty fitness store if possible. These stores will have the best equipment for the money. Delivery and setup are key when buying a multistation gym. Make sure that the store provides these services. The installation is important from a standpoint of both the operation and safety of the unit. Most stores will charge for installation, and that's OK. You need this done correctly.

Determine Your Space Allotment

I converted my garage into a workout studio, complete with rubber flooring, mirrors, and all the equipment I need for myself and my clients. Right next to the garage is my basketball court. I cannot begin to tell you how much I love and value my workout studio. I definitely created my own excuse-proof environment—which is one of the beauties of home exercising. With your gym right under your roof, it's hard to talk yourself out of working out!

Where do you plan to set up your home fitness facility? In a spare bedroom? A portion of your office? Your garage? Somewhere outdoors? Perhaps you are short on space and plan to put your cardio machine next to your bed. (That's actually a great idea. You wake up and are immediately reminded to exercise!)

You may not have a spare bedroom. You may not want to convert the garage. Perhaps you have only a small space in which to work out and must store your equipment away after use. This is perfectly fine and workable. There are functional exercise options, no matter how much room you have to work with.

Just remember to take measurements of your space before you go shopping. Below are suggested equipment units for different space configurations:

10×12-foot converted bedroom
- Multistation home gym
- Tubing
- Medicine balls
- Treadmill or elliptical trainer
- Dumbbells with an A-frame storage rack
- Flat to incline bench
- Stretch mat and stability ball

15×15-foot garage
- Treadmill or elliptical trainer
- Multistation home gym
- Stationary bike
- Heavy bag (for boxing)
- Dumbbells and a horizontal storage rack
- Tubing
- Medicine balls
- Stretch mat and stability ball
- Step-up unit

5×8-foot space next to a bed or desk
- Treadmill, elliptical trainer, stepper, or stationary bike
- Dumbbells
- Tubing
- Medicine balls
- Small multistation gym unit or fold-up gym unit

Your driveway
- Dumbbells and tubing
- Jump rope
- Medicine balls
- Step-up unit

Small apartment
- Fold-up treadmill or stationary bike
- Dumbbells and tubing
- Medicine balls
- Chin-up bar installed into wall
- Small multistation gym unit

Backyard
- Self-marked walking or running track
- Dumbbells and tubing
- Medicine balls
- Sports equipment such as basketballs, baseball and mitt, football, or heavy bag for boxing

At work
- Fold-up treadmill or stationary bike
- Jump rope
- Step-up unit
- Dumbbells and tubing
- Medicine balls
- Folding workout bench

Determine Your Budget

How much are you willing to spend on your home fitness facility? You can pay $30,000 for state-of-the-art equipment or pick up a $15 jump rope and a couple of pieces of resistance tubing. Either extreme is effective for accomplishing your weight and fat loss goals and maintaining a level of top-grade fitness. Here are some suggested facilities for sample budgets:

$20–$25
- Resistance tubing (two pieces at different resistance levels)

$40–$50
- Jump rope
- Resistance tubing (two pieces at different resistance levels)

$30–$150

- Step-up unit
- Exercise video or DVD
- Resistance tubing (three pieces at different resistance levels)
- Two pairs of dumbbell free weights
- Medicine ball

$100–$300

- Three to five pairs of dumbbell free weights
- Workout bench
- Jump rope or step-up unit
- Exercise video or DVD
- Resistance tubing (three pieces at different resistance levels)
- Medicine ball

$1,000–$2,000

- Treadmill, stationary bike, or elliptical trainer
- Four to six pairs of dumbbell free weights
- Resistance tubing (three pieces at different resistance levels)
- Stability ball
- Stretching mat
- Medicine ball

The following exercise equipment can range in price from $500 to $5,000, depending on size and quality.

- Treadmills and elliptical trainers
- Stair climbers
- Stationary bicycles, both upright and recumbent
- Rowing machines
- Cross-country ski machines
- Multistation gyms

Get Moving at Home Today

The benefits of a home fitness facility are undeniable: Forget the hassle of having to drive to the gym, change clothes, shower, dress, and drive home again just to get in that one